Basic Guide to Oral and Maxillofacial Surgery

BASIC GUIDE TO ORAL AND MAXILLOFACIAL SURGERY

Nicola Rogers

University of Bristol Dental Hospital
Bristol
UK

Cinzia Pickett

Tunbridge Wells
UK

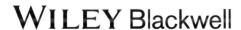

The right of Nicola Rogers and Cinzia Pickett to be identified as the authors of this work has been asserted in accordance with law.

Registered Offices: John Wiley & Sons, Inc., 111 River Street, Hoboken, NJ 07030, USA
John Wiley & Sons Ltd, The Atrium, Southern Gate, Chichester, West Sussex, PO19 8SQ, UK

Editorial Office: 9600 Garsington Road, Oxford, OX4 2DQ, UK

For details of our global editorial offices, customer services, and more information about Wiley products visit us at www.wiley.com.

Wiley also publishes its books in a variety of electronic formats and by print-on-demand. Some content that appears in standard print versions of this book may not be available in other formats.

Limit of Liability/Disclaimer of Warranty

Library of Congress Cataloging-in-Publication Data

Names: Rogers, Nicola, 1962 author. | Pickett, Cinzia, 1973 author.
Title: Basic guide to oral and maxillofacial surgery / Nikki Rogers, Cinzia
    Pickett.
Description: Hoboken, NJ : John Wiley & Sons Inc., 2017. | Includes
    bibliographical references and index.
Identifiers: LCCN 2017000446 (print) | LCCN 2017001692 (ebook) | ISBN
    9781118925072 (pbk.) | ISBN 9781118925065 (Adobe PDF) | ISBN 9781118925058
    (ePub)
Subjects: | MESH: Oral Surgical Procedures–nursing | Dental Assistants
Classification: LCC RK60.5 (print) | LCC RK60.5 (ebook) | NLM WU 600 | DDC
    617.6/01–dc23
LC record available at https://lccn.loc.gov/2017000446

Cover image: © MedicalRF.com/Gettyimages
Cover design by Wiley

Set in 10/12.5pt, SabonLTStd by SPi Global, Chennai, India

10 9 8 7 6 5 4 3 2 1

Contents

How to use this book

This book is a basic guide to maxillofacial surgery, and has been written with dental nurses in mind. It could however be used by other members of the dental team as a self-explanatory resource.

It has been compiled in order that after reading this any dental nurse, whether working in a dental practice or a specialist maxillofacial unit, would have a clear appreciation of their role during the procedures that fall under the umbrella of maxillofacial surgery. It has been written in a user-friendly manner to aid student dental nurses preparing to sit the National Examining Board for Dental Nurses' National Diploma in Dental Nursing.

There is no intention of instructing/criticising clinicians or any professionals on their role in the clinical environment, which has only been explained to further the knowledge of dental nurses throughout this book. Any offence is entirely unintended and apologies are tendered for any perceived affront. The contents of this book should not be used for diagnostic purposes.

Dental nurses are subsequently reminded/warned that on no account should they undertake any duty that is solely the province of any other General Dental Council or Health Care Professional.

Acknowledgements

To my husband David, whom I am very proud for his own personal achievements, for the love, perseverance and continual support he has shown whilst I have been co-writing this book. He is one of the most inspirational men I know and without him I wouldn't achieve the things I do.

To my son Sean, for the man he has become and his partner Zoe for the most precious gifts, our wonderful grandchildren Elsie and Lochlan.

To my parents Nigel and Valerie for always being there for me, encouraging and supporting me in everything I do, especially my Father who has constantly given his time to reading and helping me correct the chapters I have written. He is the other inspirational man in my life.

Finally I could not forget Cinzia who co-wrote this book for her support, commitment and dedication along with Wiley-Blackwell for publishing our vision.

Photographs by David Rogers courtesy of Bristol Dental Hospital.

Nicola Rogers

Writing this book has been a journey which began as a simple idea. That journey has been an incredible experience, the course of which has led me to develop a deep sense of gratitude to so many people. I am truly thankful to all of them for their combined help and support which cannot be adequately measured or expressed.

Paramount among them, however, are my friend and co-author Nicola, for her excellence in everything; our publisher Wiley-Blackwell for making the idea a reality; and my family, particularly my husband Matthew and our children Scott and Rachel for being so utterly wonderful.

Cinzia Pickett

Chapter 1

Introduction

Basic Guide to Oral and Maxillofacial Surgery, First Edition. Nicola Rogers and Cinzia Pickett.
© 2017 John Wiley & Sons Ltd. Published 2017 by John Wiley & Sons Ltd.

LEARNING OUTCOMES

At the end of this chapter you should have an understanding of:

1. Where maxillofacial surgery is carried out and by whom.
2. The procedures that are included under the umbrella of maxillofacial surgery.
3. Why maxillofacial surgery is undertaken.
4. The members of the dental team that make up the maxillofacial team.
5. The referral system.
6. The legal aspects associated with the provision of maxillofacial procedures.

INTRODUCTION

Maxillofacial surgery forms an appreciable part of daily practice for the non-specialist dentist. Some restrict their practice to straightforward extractions while others undertake a wide range of surgical procedures associated with the jaws, teeth and soft tissues. Many refer to this practice as minor oral surgery. There are specialist centres and departments within local dental and general hospitals where clinicians are committed to procedures that come under the umbrella of maxillofacial surgery. These include:

- Straightforward extractions.
- Surgical removal of impacted and broken-down teeth.
- Surgical removal of retained roots.
- Biopsies, which involve a sample of tissue being removed and sent for diagnosis to confirm or eliminate a diagnosis.
- Exposure of impacted canines for patients undergoing orthodontic treatment.
- Frenectomy, which is where either the labial or lingual frenulum is released.

- The removal of cysts.
- Alveolectomies, undertaken prior to dentures being supplied to a patient. This involves the smoothing off of the alveolar ridge.
- Performing apicectomies where other root treatments have failed or it is impossible for them to be carried out. In dentistry an apicectomy comes under the auspices of endodontic treatments; however, as they involve raising a flap, it is classed as a surgical procedure.
- Removal of tumours.
- Reconstruction of the face following trauma or removal of facial tissues and structures.
- Cosmetic treatments such as a face lift, rhinoplasty (the correction and reconstruction of the nose) or otoplasty (ears that stick out), commonly known as bat ears.
- Orthognathic surgery, which is where surgical intervention is undertaken to correct jaw discrepancies.

For a clinician to undertake the last four procedures he/she must be dually qualified in dentistry and medicine.

The reason these procedures may be undertaken can be attributed to disease, accidental injury, congenital malformation, periodontal problems and caries. These treatments can be carried out with the use of local anaesthetic, either on its own or in combination with a form of conscious sedation, or a general anaesthetic, thereby involving many team members.

The maxillofacial team comprises the following members:

- Consultant.
- Registrar.
- Oral surgeons.
- Senior house officers.
- Dental nurses.
- Anaesthetists.
- Recovery nurses who are state registered, with anaesthetic training.

When patients are being treated for cancerous lesions, a multi-disciplinary team approach involves additional team members. These are:

- Oncologists (a specialist who treats cancerous lesions).
- Radiologists (a specialist in interpreting images of the body).
- Microbiologists and pathologists (who study micro-organisms and how they affect the human body).
- Specialist head and neck nurses (registered general nurses).
- Macmillan nurses (registered general nurses who specialise in the care of oncology patients).

- Speech and language therapists (specialists who are trained to aid patients with their speech).
- Dieticians (a specialist in nutrition or dietetics).

PATIENT REFERRAL

Patients are referred to specialist units and departments within local dental and general hospitals where maxillofacial surgery is undertaken. Reasons for referring patients can include the following:

- It is thought that the patient will be managed more appropriately due to the complexity of the treatment required, or their medical history.
- The patient's general dental practitioner requires a specialist opinion.
- The patient's general dental practitioner does not offer the treatment the patient requires.
- The general dental practitioner offers the treatment the patient requires, but does not offer the method of pain and anxiety control the patient requests.

When a general dental practitioner refers a patient for maxillofacial treatment they must provide a referral letter which will, as a minimum, contain the following information:

- Patient personal details: name, address, telephone number and date of birth.
- Patient medical history.
- The presenting dental problem.
- The reason for the referral.
- The name and contact details of the referring general dental practitioner.
- Any radiographs taken.

Many specialist units and departments within local dental and general hospitals have forms that can be completed to make the referral process easier. If the general dental practitioner or the patient's general practitioner suspects a cancerous lesion, they can use a fast track referral form. Some forms request additional information to that listed above in order to allow the member of the maxillofacial surgery team assessing the referral form/letter to assign a suitable time frame for the patient to be seen. Once this has been undertaken, an appointment will be sent to the patient for a consultation. Once the patient has been seen by the specialist unit or departments within local dental and general hospitals, an outcome letter is sent to the referring practitioner. This will contain a diagnosis and whether the patient has been or will be treated by a member of the maxillofacial team, or are being returned into the care of a general dental practitioner or general practitioner for ongoing treatment and care. Any dental radiographs furbished by the general dental practitioner will be returned.

LEGAL ASPECTS ASSOCIATED WITH MAXILLOFACIAL SURGERY

The legal aspects associated with maxillofacial surgery are no different from any other specialist field within medicine and dentistry. On a daily basis, the maxillofacial surgeon must consider the following legal and ethical issues:

- Negligence.
- Confidentiality.
- Consent.
- Accusations of assault.

Negligence

For a member of the maxillofacial team to be negligent, they will have acted outside the law and/or will have undertaken treatment that is not satisfactory. All members of the maxillofacial team have a duty of care to ensure that every patient is treated safely, with a high standard of care being provided. Good communication with patients and the rest of the maxillofacial team is therefore paramount to avoid any misunderstandings. The taking of consent is mandatory, as this will provide documentation of which treatments were agreed and those that were not. Well-kept dental notes will provide a history of the patient's past, present and future treatment. All members of the maxillofacial team must be trained for their area of responsibility and must not work outside that remit and scope of practice. A safe clinical environment should be provided for all, with any equipment being serviced at recommended intervals to avoid any accidents or incidents.

Confidentiality

When a patient provides the maxillofacial team with any information about themselves, they expect it to be kept confidential. This means that all members of the maxillofacial team must not divulge any information relating to patients. They must also ensure that all precautions are taken to prevent any information being divulged unintentionally. All patient information must be kept secure as patients discuss delicate issues with the maxillofacial team/clinician pertinent to their treatment. Patient information cannot be released without the consent of the patient. However, there are exceptional situations where patient information can be disclosed without requesting the patient's consent. These include:

- Where it would benefit them (e.g. their health was at risk).
- Where it was considered that a serious crime was imminent.
- In the interests of the general public.

If any of these situations occur the patient's consent should ideally still be sought and, if not given, only minimal information should be released. Patients should always be aware that their information may be shared with other healthcare professionals. Confidentiality extends after the death of a patient.

Consent

When taken, consent can help to protect the maxillofacial surgeon from complaints, claims and charges as documentary evidence will be available of all discussions held. Consent is a process where one person grants another permission to undertake something such as maxillofacial surgery. It is given once the patient consenting is aware of what is going to happen, and they can withdraw their consent at any time. Consent can be obtained in any of several forms. It can be written, verbal or a compliant action. Obtaining written consent from a patient is a must for all maxillofacial surgery, as complications may occur. Forms are available for use and, when completed, will contain the patient's personal details as well as the practice details. It must be completed in ink without any abbreviations being used. The age of the patient and the capacity of a patient to consent will determine which consent form is to be completed. It will be signed by both parties, with a copy being given to the patient. If the patient does not want a copy, then this must be recorded in the notes.

Only the member of the maxillofacial team qualified to undertake the proposed treatment can take consent from a patient. Consent should be obtained in a quiet, private area to maintain patient confidentiality. All aspects of treatment will be discussed and the patient must be allowed to ask questions. Dental nurses cannot take consent, but best practice would be to ensure that consent is in place prior to maxillofacial surgery. For consent to be valid, a patient must have the mental capacity to give consent and give it voluntarily. They must be able to understand and retain the information given, contemplate it and come to a decision themselves. The maxillofacial team must describe to the patient all aspects relating to treatment which must include the advantages and disadvantages, any associated risks, alternative treatments, time frames of the proposed treatment and associated costs. Consent forms can vary according to the clinical environment; many hospitals and trusts utilise the NHS consent forms, therefore providing standardisation.

Assault

Any maxillofacial surgery undertaken without a patient's consent is regarded as assault, and the member of the team who undertook such treatment could therefore be accountable for any implications arising. As patients can make allegations of assault, maxillofacial surgeons must always be chaperoned with consent in place.

RECORD KEEPING

The maintenance of a patient's dental records/notes is paramount with contemporaneous notes being beneficial to both the patient and the maxillofacial surgeon. Failure to maintain these could lead to serious implications for both the patient and the maxillofacial surgeon as they provide personal details pertaining to a patient and a chronological account of the treatment the patient has received or any that is pending. They will include details of any discussions that have been held, including those during the consent process. It must be remembered that records of the patient extend to photographs, radiographs and study models and that all must be correctly processed, only used for the purpose for which they were intended and disposed of correctly when no longer required.

Medical, dental and social histories must all be documented and considered by the maxillofacial surgeon so that the patient receives the best possible care. Failure to ensure this could mean that patient care is compromised, which could lead to litigation.

Medical history

It is essential for a medical history to be taken in order to provide individual care, tailored to the patient's needs. This is usually gained through a questionnaire which asks set questions pertaining to any illnesses the patient has or has previously suffered. It will contain questions relating to any medication the patient takes, both prescribed and non-prescribed, including recreational. Other information requested will be family history, previous operations with or without a general anaesthetic, any recent travel abroad, and drinking and smoking habits. From this a clear picture of the patient's medical status can be formed before providing any maxillofacial treatment. A patient's medical history must be updated every time they attend for treatment in order to establish if there have been any changes; if so, their impact on the patient's treatment plan must be assessed and the treatment plan modified if necessary.

Dental history

To establish the patient's dental history, expectations and attitudes towards their dental health, the maxillofacial surgeon will discuss with the patient their previous experiences and dental history as well as the presenting dental problem. Past methods of pain and anxiety control used will also be explored to establish if anything other than a local anaesthetic needs to be considered. All of these are important as they could be detrimental to effective management. A clinical examination with or without radiographs will provide a picture of the patient's dental health and their motivation in maintaining good oral health.

Social history

This history is as important as the others, as the maxillofacial surgeon has a duty of care to ensure that the patient will be adequately cared for at home. This is particularly pertinent when the patient is receiving treatment with intravenous, transmucosal or oral sedation. As consent is required for maxillofacial surgery, the maxillofacial surgeon has to be sure the patient is competent to give this; if not, another means of acquiring consent must be found. The cost of maxillofacial surgery has to be deliberated and discussed with the patient in order to determine whether they can afford to proceed or not. If not, other ways of handling their dental care have to be explored.

INTRODUCTION

Chapter 2

Anatomy of the head, neck and skull

INTRODUCTION

As part of multi-disciplinary team, knowledge of the structures of the head, neck and skull is needed. Along with a basic understanding of conditions and lesions that patients may present within the maxillofacial outpatients department, such knowledge forms an important base for the dental care professional.

A HEALTHY MOUTH

It is important to understand the presentation of a healthy mouth in order to recognise abnormalities. When the maxillofacial surgeon looks in a patient's mouth they examine the teeth for signs of caries, the gingiva for any indications of periodontal disease and the oral mucosa and tongue to ensure its presentation is normal. In a healthy mouth the teeth should sit firmly in the

Basic Guide to Oral and Maxillofacial Surgery, First Edition. Nicola Rogers and Cinzia Pickett.
© 2017 John Wiley & Sons Ltd. Published 2017 by John Wiley & Sons Ltd.

alveolar bone, being attached to it by the periodontal ligaments. The bone and periodontal ligaments are covered by the gingiva lining the alveolar ridge. The gingiva is attached to the neck of the tooth at the junctional epithelium with the gingival crevice being no more than 2 mm. The gingivae is pink in colour, having an orange peel effect with a tight gingival cuff around the tooth. There should be no bleeding on probing and, sub-gingivally, the periodontal ligaments and alveolar bone should be intact. Any examination that highlights disease will be investigated and treated accordingly.

ANATOMICAL TERMS

In order to describe the position of a structure relative to another, the following terms are often used in dentistry:

- **Anterior** – In front of.
- **Posterior** – Behind.
- **Superior** – Above.
- **Inferior** – Below.
- **Medial** – Towards the mid-line.
- **Lateral** – Away from the mid-line or to one side of.

ANATOMY OF THE SKULL

The skull (Figures 2.1 and 2.2) has two defined areas: the cranium and facial. There are eight bones that make up the cranium. The single bones are the frontal, occipital, sphenoid and ethmoid and the paired bones are the parietal and temporal.

Bones of the neurocranium

Frontal
Part of the cranium, this single bone forms the forehead, known as the frontal eminences. Within the frontal bone lie the frontal sinuses. The frontal bone consists of many landmark areas such as the superciliary arches, supraorbital margins, glabella and nasion.

Superciliary arch
The area of thickened bone which lies beneath the eyebrows.

Supraorbital margins
The area below the superciliary arches round to the superior area of the orbits.

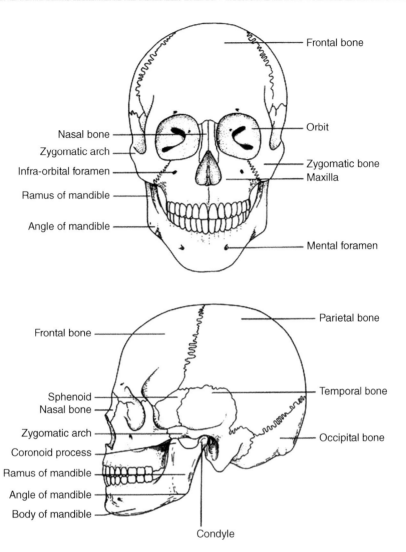

Figure 2.1 The skull. Source: Hollins, C. 2013. *Levison's Textbook for Dental Nurses*, 11th Edition, p. 231. Reproduced with permission of John Wiley & Sons.

Glabella

The area of frontal bone which joins the superciliary arches. The frontal suture can sometimes be traced on and above the glabella.

Nasion

This is the midpoint of the frontonasal suture, and is the connection between the frontal and nasal bones. The frontonasal suture is found below the frontal suture.

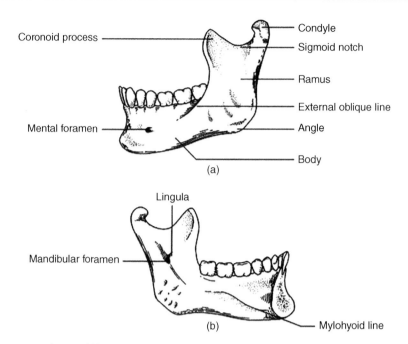

Figure 2.2 The mandible: (a) outer side and (b) inner side. Source: Hollins, C. 2013. *Levison's Textbook for Dental Nurses*, 11th Edition, p. 235. Reproduced with permission of John Wiley & Sons.

Occipital

This single bone forms the lower posterior area of the cranium. Areas of the occipital bone include the squama, foramen magnum, hypoglossal canal, occipital condyles, external occipital protuberance and external occipital crest. The following explains where they sit anatomically:

- **Squama:** The occipital squama has a curved surface and is the area above and behind the foramen magnum.
- **Forman magnum:** Oval in shape, this opening is in the lower part of the occipital bone.
- **Hypoglossal canal:** A tunnelled canal found in the base of each occipital condyle.
- **Occipital condyles:** Two bony protrusions at the base of the occipital, which articulate with the first cervical vertebrae.
- **External occipital protuberance:** This prominent, curved area of bone is found halfway between the magnum foramen and the top of the occipital bone.
- **External occipital crest:** An external crest which extends downwards from the occipital protuberance to the foramen magnum.

- **Sphenoid:** A winged-shaped bone which forms part of the external and internal neurocranium. The outer edge of the wing is located anterior to the temporal bone.

Ethmoid
This bone comprises a vertical and horizontal plate, a lateral mass (orbital plate and ethmoid sinuses) and a mid-nasal concha and crista galli. It is a complex, deeply seated bone between the nasal cavity and orbits. It forms part of the nasal septum along with the vomer; it also forms the medial aspect of the walls of the orbit and nasal cavity.

Parietal
These paired bones form a simple curved shape. The parietal bones form the superior, lateral and posterior area of the cranium.

Temporal
The temporal bones are paired, one found on each side. They form the side and base of the skull. Each single temporal bone comprises the squama, tympanic and petrous regions. The temporal bone forms part of the temporal mandibular joint. The following explains where they are positioned anatomically:

- **Squama:** A broad, flat area of the temporal bone which is found in the anterior and superior region.
- **Tympanic:** A curved plate of bone which surrounds the external auditory meatus and also forms the bony regions of this structure.
- **Petrous:** A pyramid-shaped bone at the base of the skull between the sphenoid and occipital bones.

Facial bones

The facial area of the skull consists of 14 bones. The majority of these bones are paired, with the exception of the single mandible and vomer. The paired bones are the maxilla, zygomatic, nasal, lacrimal, palatine and inferior nasal conchae.

Mandible
This bone forms the lower third of the face, and is the only movable bone within the skull as it can swing from side to side. It is made up of the following anatomical features:

- **Angle of the mandible:** This is where the ascending ramus meets the body of the mandible to form an angle.
- **Body of the mandible:** This is the main part of the mandible that extends anteriorly from the angle to the corner of the mental protuberance.

ANATOMY OF THE HEAD,
NECK AND SKULL

- **Ramus:** This area is the vertical section of the mandible that extends above the angle to join with the condyle and coronoid process.
- **Condyle:** This forms part of the temporomandibular joint and is the rounded bone that sits posteriorly at the top of the ramus.
- **Coronoid process:** This forms part of the temporomandibular joint and is the bony projection that sits anteriorly at the top of the ramus.
- **Sigmoid notch:** This is the depression in the bone that is situated between the condyle and coronoid process.
- **Mental foramen:** A foramen is a natural opening in bone which permits vessels to enter and exit. The mental foramens are found marginally below and in the region of the first and second pre-molar teeth.
- **Mental protuberance:** This bone is the prominent anterior projection of the mandible and forms the chin. The size and shape of this bone depicts the size and shape of the chin.
- **External oblique line (ridge):** An external oblique ridge extends across the external surface of the body of the mandible.
- **Mylohyoid ridge:** This bone is an attachment for the mylohyoid muscle and is an internal ridge that runs on the internal surface of the mandible.
- **Lingula:** This is a bony projection that is situated on the anterior border of the mandibular foramen to protect the mandibular nerve as it enters the mandibular foramen.
- **Genial tubercles:** These are slight prominent bones which sit just above the lower border of the mandible in the midline.

Vomer

This bone, along with the ethmoid and palatine bones, forms part of the nasal septum.

Maxilla

This bone forms the upper jaw and comprises of the following anatomical features:

- **Incisive foramen:** This is located in the anterior aspect of the palate in the region of the incisor teeth. It permits the nasopalatine nerve, also known as the long sphenopalatine, to enter into the mouth.
- **Alveolar process:** This is a ridge-like bone which is made up of sockets for the mandibular and maxillary teeth to sit in. The roots of a tooth are embedded in this process. It may be referred to as the maxillary and mandibular ridge.
- **Canine fossa:** This is a depression on the anterior surface of the maxilla, situated below the infraorbital foramen on the lateral side of the canine eminence.

- **Canine eminence:** This is a prominence in the maxillary alveolar process that covers the root of the canine teeth.

Zygomatic

This area is part of the facial skeleton that forms the cheek and the lateral wall of the orbit. It connects the cranium to the maxilla. There are three bones that support the zygomatic arch: the maxilla anteriorly; the frontal bone superiorly; and the temporal bone posteriorly. A buttressing effect is produced, which helps to support the zygomatic arch. The zygomaticofacial foramen is found at the prominence of the zygomatic bone.

Nasal

The nasal bones, of which there are two, form the structure of the nose. Varying in size and shape, the nasal bones act as an attachment for cartilage which then forms the individual's nose contours.

Lacrimal

This is the smallest and most fragile bone on the face. It is situated at the anterior medial wall of the orbit.

Palatine

The palatine bone is a concave structure which superiorly forms the base of the nasal cavity and inferiorly forms the hard palate.

Inferior nasal conchae

There are three pairs of nasal conchae. The superior and middle conchae are formed by the ethmoid bone. The inferior conchae are separate bones and form part of the lateral walls of the nasal cavity.

The orbital area

The margins and walls of the orbital area are formed by several cranium and facial bones:

- **Superior orbital margin and roof:** frontal.
- **Lateral orbital margin and anterior lateral wall:** zygomatic.
- **Lateral orbital posterior wall:** sphenoid.
- **Inferior orbital margin:** laterally zygomatic, medially maxilla.
- **Orbital floor:** maxilla.
- **Medially:** maxilla, lacrimal, ethmoid and sphenoid bones.

NERVE SUPPLY TO THE TEETH AND THEIR SURROUNDING STRUCTURES

There are twelve pairs of cranial nerves. These originate inside the skull from the brain and pass through the skull to supply the muscles and structures of the head and neck. Nerves are described as either motor, sensory or mixed. Sensory nerves transmit impulses from the sense organs (eyes, ears, etc.) to the spinal cord and the brain. Motor nerves transmit impulses from the brain and spinal cord to stimulate muscles to contract, whereas mixed nerves contain both sensory and motor fibres. In dentistry, we are concerned with only two of the cranial nerves:

1. The Vth cranial nerve, known as the trigeminal.
2. The VIIth cranial nerve, known as the facial.

Trigeminal nerve

This is the largest cranial nerve. It has a large sensory root and a smaller motor root, and divides into three branches which arise from the trigeminal ganglion inside the skull:

- **Ophthalmic division:** This is a sensory nerve that supplies the forehead, top of the nose and upper eyelids.
- **Maxillary division:** This is a sensory nerve that supplies the upper jaw, teeth and the middle part of the facial skin (Table 2.1).
- **Mandibular division:** This is a sensory and motor nerve, which supplies the skin over the temple, the muscles, the lower jaw and teeth, the front of the tongue and lower lip. The motor nerve for the muscles of mastication is part of the mandibular nerve (Table 2.2).

The maxillary and mandibular nerves are anaesthetised during maxillofacial surgery in order to provide pain-free treatment.

Maxillary division

After leaving the trigeminal ganglion, the nerve passes through the skull via the foramen rotundum in the greater wing of the sphenoid. It passes through the upper part of the pterygopalatine fossa and enters the orbit through the inferior orbital fissure.

In the pterygopalatine fossa, it gives off three branches:

- **The zygomatic nerve:** This enters the zygomatic bone and sends branches to the temporal fossa, the skin of the cheek, via the zygomatic-facial foramen.

Table 2.1 Nerve supply to the maxillary division

Teeth and their surrounding tissue	Nerve
8, 7 distal aspect of the 6 and the buccal gingivae	Posterior superior alveolar dental
Mesial aspect of the 6, 5 and 4 and the buccal gingivae	Middle superior alveolar dental
3, 2, 1 and the buccal gingivae	Anterior superior alveolar dental
Palatal gingivae of 1–3	Nasopalatine/long sphenopalatine
Palatal gingivae of 3–8	Greater palatine nerve
Soft palate	Lesser palatine nerve

Table 2.2 Nerve supply to the mandibular division

Teeth and their surrounding tissue	Nerve
Teeth 1–8	Inferior dental
Buccal gingivae 1–5	Long buccal
Buccal gingivae 6–8	Mental
Lingual gingivae 1–8, anterior 2/3 of the tongue and floor of mouth	Lingual nerve

ANATOMY OF THE HEAD, NECK AND SKULL

- **The superior alveolar dental nerve:** Branches from this nerve pass into the posterior surface of the maxilla to run in the canals of the wall of the sinus on their way to join the middle superior alveolar branches. The **posterior superior alveolar nerve** supplies the third and second molar, the distal root of the first molar and the buccal gingivae of these teeth. Within the infraorbital canal, the maxillary nerve gives off the middle superior and anterior superior alveolar nerve. The **middle superior alveolar nerve** supplies the premolars, the mesiobuccal root of the first molar and the buccal gingivae of these teeth. When this nerve is missing, the supply is from the posterior superior alveolar nerve. The **anterior superior alveolar nerve** supplies the incisors, canine and labial gingivae of these teeth. The sphenopalatine ganglion acts as a relay station which is a circular enlargement of nervous tissue suspended from the maxillary nerve close to its origin. It gives rise to the greater and lesser palatine and naso palatine nerves.
- **The naso palatine nerve** supplies the palatal gingivae of the incisors and part of the canine and active, or part of the mucous membrane of the hard palate.

The **greater palatine nerve** supplies the palatal gingivae of the canine, premolars and molars and mucous membrane of the hard palate. The **lesser palatine nerve** supplies the soft palate

The maxillary nerve finally passes through the infraorbital foramen on the front of the maxilla to supply the skin and mucous membrane of the lower eyelid, cheek, nose and upper lip.

Mandibular division

The mandibular nerve arises at the trigeminal ganglion. It passes down from the base of the skull on the inner surface of the ramus of the mandible, between the ;medial and lateral pterygoid muscles, and divides into two main branches. The anterior branch supplies the muscles of mastication and the posterior branch, which gives off:

- **The inferior dental nerve:** This nerve enters the mandible via the mandibular foramen which is situated on the inner surface of the ramus next to the lingula (a small bony projection). The inferior dental nerve travels along the mandibular canal below the apices of the teeth, supplying sensation to the lower teeth, and then forwards to the mental foramen. This then gives off the mental nerve.
- **The mental nerve:** This branch of the inferior dental nerve emerges from the mandibular canal via the mental foramen which is situated below the apices of the premolars. It supplies the skin and mucous membrane of the chin and lower lip and periodontal membranes of the premolars. If anaesthetic solution is passed into the foramen itself, the premolars, canines and incisors will also be anaesthetised (mental block).
- **The long buccal nerve:** This nerve supplies the buccal gingivae of the molars.
- **Lingual nerve:** This nerve supplies the lingual gingivae of all the lower teeth as well as the anterior two-thirds of the tongue and floor of the mouth. When this nerve is anaesthetised, the tongue is also affected.

Facial nerve

The facial nerve is mainly a motor nerve which supplies most of the muscles that move the mouth and face. It also supplies some fibres to the anterior two-thirds of the tongue with taste sensation. When this nerve is damaged or affected by disease the muscles cannot work properly; this causes drooping of the face, known as Bell's or facial palsy.

MAJOR BLOOD VESSELS OF THE HEAD AND NECK

The major blood vessels within the head and neck run adjacent to the nerve supply within that area known as neurovascular bundles. They carry oxygenated blood to the head and neck and drain the deoxygenated blood. The common carotid arteries carry the oxygenated blood and jugular veins carry deoxygenated blood to the superior vena cava. The main vessels are:

- **External carotid artery:** It divides into six branches to supply oxygenated blood to the external areas of the head and neck.
- **Internal carotid artery:** This artery supplies oxygenated blood to the internal areas of the head, forehead, brain and eyes. It does not supply any structures within the neck.
- **External jugular vein:** This vein takes deoxygenated blood from the external regions of the neurocranium.
- **Internal jugular vein:** This major vessel takes deoxygenated blood from the brain and most of the head and neck.

SALIVARY GLANDS

Within the mouth there are three large, paired glands called the major salivary glands (Figure 2.3; Table 2.3), known as:

- The parotid.
- The submandibular.
- The sublingual.

There are also 800–1000 minor salivary glands within the mucous membranes of the lips, cheeks, palate and tongue. Each gland consists of a group

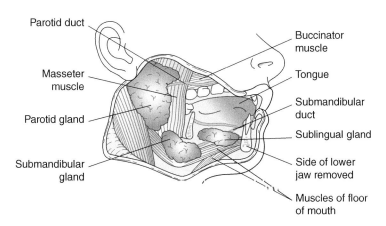

Figure 2.3 Major salivary glands. Source: Hollins, C. 2012. *Basic Guide to Anatomy and Physiology for Dental Care Professionals*, p. 168. Reproduced with permission of John Wiley & Sons.

Table 2.3 Salivary glands

Salivary gland	Salivary duct	Shape	Opening within the mouth	Additional information
Parotid	Stenson's	Pyramidal	Mid-line beside the lingual fraenum	The gland swells in cases of mumps
Submandibular	Wharton's	Walnut	Buccal sulcus opposite the first and second molar tooth	Stones or calculus can be found in the duct as it runs uphill
Sublingual	8–20 excretory ducts		Floor of the mouth just behind the submandibular duct	A blockage may occur in one of these ducts due to a cyst rannula leading to a unilateral swelling in the floor of the mouth, which is bluish in colour and full of mucous

of cells called acini; each acinus is formed by a group of cells surrounded by a small central canal. These canals link to form a main duct through which the saliva is passed into the mouth.

MUSCLES OF THE HEAD AND NECK

The muscles of the head and neck are accountable for moving the head along with a range of movements that include the eyes, mastication and facial expression. They are grouped as:

- Muscles of mastication (Table 2.4).
- Muscles of facial expression (Table 2.5).
- Muscles of the tongue (Table 2.6).
- Suprahyoid muscles (Table 2.7).

Nerve supply to the muscles of the head and neck

The muscles of mastication are supplied by the mandibular division of the fifth cranial nerve (Vth), known as the trigeminal nerve. The muscles of facial expression are supplied by the seventh cranial nerve (VIIth), known as the facial nerve. The muscles of the tongue are supplied by the mandibular division of the trigeminal nerve. The suprahyoid muscles are supplied by both the fifth (V) and seventh (VII) cranial nerve.

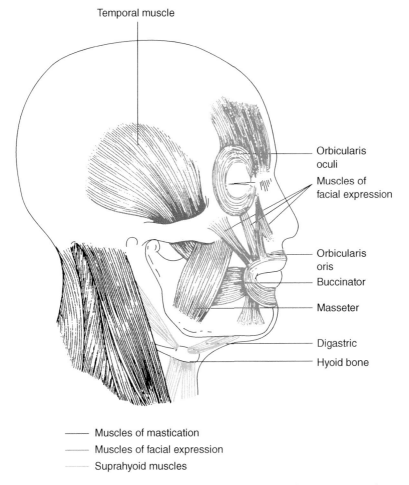

Temporal muscle

Orbicularis oculi

Muscles of facial expression

Orbicularis oris

Buccinator

Masseter

Digastric

Hyoid bone

—— Muscles of mastication
—— Muscles of facial expression
—— Suprahyoid muscles

Figure 2.4 Oral musculature. Source: Hollins, C. 2012. *Basic Guide to Anatomy and Physiology for Dental Care Professionals*, p. 125. Reproduced with permission of John Wiley & Sons.

Muscles of mastication

The muscles of mastication (Figure 2.4 and Table 2.4) control mouth closure and the action of chewing. They are attached from the cranium to the mandible. On each side of the skull there are four muscles of mastication:

- The masseter.
- The temporalis.
- The medial pterygoid.
- The lateral pterygoid.

ANATOMY OF THE HEAD, NECK AND SKULL

Table 2.4 Muscles of mastication

Muscle	Shape	Origin	Insertion	Action
Masseter	Square	Zygomatic arch	External surface of the angle of the mandible and the body of the ramus of the mandible	Closes the mouth
Temporalis	Large fan	Temporal bone	Coronoid process	Closes the mouth
Medial pterygoid	Square	Medial pterygoid plate of the sphenoid bone	Inner surface of the ramus of the mandible	Lifts and closes the mouth
Lateral pterygoid	Short cone	Lateral pterygoid plate of the sphenoid bone	Anterior aspect of the condyle and the capsule of the temporal mandibular joint	If both contract the mandible moves forward. If one contracts the mandible moves from side to side.

Table 2.5 Muscles of facial expression

Name	Origin	Insertion	Function
Orbicularis oris	Encircles the mouth joining the buccinator muscle	It is NOT attached to bone	Closes and protrudes the lips, pressing them together. Tightens and thins the lips, rolling them in between the teeth and thrusting them outwards
Orbicularis oculi	The medial part of the orbit running around the eye via the upper eye lids	None	Closes the eyelids
Buccinator	From the alveolar process of the maxilla and mandible	Into the fibres of the orbicularis oris at the angle of the mouth	Helps maintain a bolus of food in the mouth during chewing and swallowing. It acts to compress the cheeks to the teeth.

Muscles of facial expression

The muscles of facial expression (Table 2.5) produce a variety of movement and facial expressions. When they contract they result in skin movement. They are like elastic sheets that are stretched in layers over the cranium, facial bones, the openings they form, cartilage, fat and other tissues of the head. They are known as:

- **Orbicularis oris:** sphincter muscle around the mouth.
- **Orbicularis oculi:** sphincter muscle of the eye.
- **Buccinator:** a thin, flat muscle on the side of the face.

Muscles of the tongue

The tongue is a very muscular mobile organ (Table 2.6) associated with taste, chewing, speaking and predominately deglutition (swallowing). It lies in the floor of the mouth. The posterior aspect of the tongue is situated in the throat, being attached to the floor of the mouth with the anterior aspect (two-thirds) lying within the oral cavity. It is the latter that is mobile.

The surfaces of the tongue are:

- Dorsum (upper surface).
- Tip.
- Root (deep attachment in the pharynx).
- Inferior.

The muscles of the tongue are divided into two groups:

- Extrinsic.
- Intrinsic.

Table 2.6 Muscles of the tongue

Muscle	Position	Action
Extrinsic: hyoglossus; geniohyoid; genioglossus; styloglossus; and palatoglossus	Outside the body of the tongue	Moves the tongue and alters its shape
Intrinsic	Within the body of the tongue	Alters the shape of the tongue

ANATOMY OF THE HEAD, NECK AND SKULL

Suprahyoid muscles

The suprahyoid muscles (Table 2.7) control the opening of the mouth and swallowing. They are attached to bone and structures in the neck. There are anterior and posterior muscles. The anterior are known as:

- Mylohoid.
- Geniohyoid.
- Anterior digastric.

  The posterior are known as:

- Stylohyoid.
- Posterior digastric.

Table 2.7 Suprahyoid muscles

Muscle	Origin	Insertion	Action
Mylohoid	Mylohoid line	Hyoid bone	Opens the mouth and, when swallowing, lifts the hyoid bone and larynx
Geniohyoid	Genial tubercules	Hyoid bone	Opens the mouth and, when swallowing, lifts the hyoid bone and larynx
Anterior digastric	Hyoid bone	Mental symphysis	Opens the mouth by pulling the jaw down; when swallowing it lifts the hyoid bone and larynx
Stylohyoid	Styloid process	Hyoid bone	When swallowing it lifts the hyoid bone and larynx
Posterior digastric	Mastoid process	Hyoid bone	When swallowing it lifts the hyoid bone and larynx

Chapter 3

Pain and anxiety control

LEARNING OUTCOMES

At the end of this chapter you should have an understanding of:

1. Why pain and anxiety control is important.
2. The different methods of pain and anxiety control used.

INTRODUCTION

Managing patients' pain and anxiety control commences at the assessment stage of an appointment where the clinician undertakes a medical, dental and social history. The three histories are equally important as this gives the clinician an understanding of the patient's anxiety levels, preferences, any medical conditions and/or medications taken. From this information the clinician can correctly plan a patient's treatment taking into account these factors so that the patient will be safely treated in the dental surgery, along with their pain relief being individualised for them.

In their *Maintaining Standards* booklet, the General Dental Council have outlined a logical progression for pain and anxiety control stating that the mainstay/starting point of managing a patient's pain relief is by using a local anaesthetic.

To appreciate pain and anxiety control methods used, it is important to understand the nerve supply to the maxilla and mandible along with their surrounding structures as discussed in Chapter 2, as well as the following terminology used:

- **Analgesia:** the absence of pain without loss of consciousness.

Basic Guide to Oral and Maxillofacial Surgery, First Edition. Nicola Rogers and Cinzia Pickett.
© 2017 John Wiley & Sons Ltd. Published 2017 by John Wiley & Sons Ltd.

- **Anaesthesia:** loss of all sensations, including pain, with or without loss of consciousness.
- **Anaesthetic:** an agent which produces anaesthesia.
- **General anaesthesia:** the loss of sensation produced by putting a patient to sleep, thereby preventing reception of pain by the brain.
- **Local anaesthesia:** the loss of feeling or sensation in some part of the body due to nerve impulse blockage, by use of drugs preventing conduction of stimuli along a nerve.
- **Conscious sedation:** the administration of sedatives or dissociative agents with or without a local anaesthetic to help the patient accept dental treatment. At all times the patient remains conscious.

If a patient does not receive enough pain relief when undertaking maxillofacial surgery procedures they will be uncomfortable as they will experience pain. This could lead to an uncooperative patient which could have a detrimental effect on their oral health care as they may not attend the dentist in the future due to the experience.

LOCAL ANAESTHETIC

A local anaesthetic is administered when any procedure involves soft tissues, enabling a patient to endure the dental treatment due to being pain free. Pressure and vibrations can still be felt and quite often these sensations are interpreted by the patient as pain; good patient management is therefore important. By providing the patient with a local anaesthetic the area administered will be numb, making it insensitive to pain without affecting their other senses. On occasions a clinician may apply a topical anaesthetic gel (Figure 3.1) to slightly de-sensitise the area being injected, thereby making the administration of the local anaesthetic more comfortable for the patient. Clinicians must appreciate the concentration and effects of the local anaesthetic they are administering to avoid reaching the maximum toxic dose. This will naturally vary from patient to patient depending upon their weight. For example, if septocaine (commonly referred to as articaine; Figure 3.1) was being administered and the patient weighed 70 kg, the maximum amount of cartridges that could be administered is 7.

How local anaesthetics work

Painful sensations from dental structures are directed to the brain along specific nerve pathways, where they are interpreted as pain. An administration

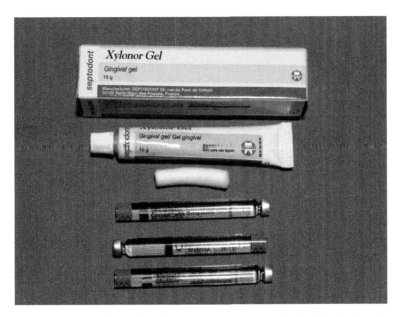

Figure 3.1 Topical anaesthetic gel and anaesthetic cartridges: articaine 4% solution with epinephrine 1:100,000 lignocaine (xylocaine) 2% and adrenaline 1 in 80,000; and prilocaine (citanest) 3% and octopressin (felypressin).

of a local anaesthetic around any of these nerves or their branches temporarily prevents them from conveying painful messages to the brain. As previously explained however, pressure and vibrations can still be felt. After a while the effect of the local anaesthetic will wear off and the nerve impulses return to normal. A dental injection will be administered into an area which is richly supplied with blood vessels. This means that the local anaesthetic solution is rapidly absorbed into the blood stream. Due to the rapidity in which anaesthetic agents are removed from the injected area, plain anaesthetic such as lignocaine (xylocaine) (Figure 3.1) will not last long enough for most dental procedures; to overcome this, a vasoconstrictor is added to the solution to prolong the duration of action.

Vasoconstrictors

A vasoconstrictor will produce vasoconstriction of the vessels in the area where the local anaesthetic has been administered, thereby reducing the blood flow to prolong anaesthesia. They also reduce bleeding, which is a useful function during maxillofacial surgery due to these being bloodletting procedures. There are two types of vasoconstrictors used:

- **Adrenaline:** This vasoconstrictor is naturally occurring in the body, but is not suitable for all patients as it can affect the heart rate and blood pressure.

- **Octopressin:** This vasoconstrictor is not suitable for pregnant patients as it has the ability to mimic the hormone oxytosin which stimulates the uterus during labour; if administered, it could result in premature labour.

It must be remembered that the choice of local anaesthetic to be used which contains a vasoconstrictor would be the responsibility of the treating clinician for each patient.

Equipment required to administer a local anaesthetic

The following equipment is required to administer a local anaesthetic:

- **A sterile self-aspirating syringe (Figure 3.2):** This type of syringe is used to avoid the anaesthetic being injected into a blood vessel. If, upon administration, blood flowed into the cartridge the clinician should stop administration and reposition the needle until the blood disappeared.
- **A sterile disposable needle:** Either a gauge 27 (long) (Figure 3.2) or gauge 30 or 31 (short and shorter) (Figure 3.2) depending upon the clinician's choice and the site of the injection.
- The local anaesthetic cartridge chosen by the clinician.
- A topical anaesthetic and cotton wool roll for application if the clinician chooses.

Topical anaesthetic

Topical anaesthetics are applied to the appropriate area for a few minutes prior to an injection being administered to relieve discomfort. They take about 2 minutes to work and last for approximately 10 minutes. They are available as a gel or spray for dental use and commonly contain an anaesthetic agent such as lidocaine or benzocaine. Some clinicians may choose to use a flavoured topical gel, which is more easily tolerated by children.

Local anaesthetic presentation

The local anaesthetic agent/solution is supplied in glass cartridges which have a rubber diaphragm at one end and a rubber bung at the other. Each cartridge contains either 1.8 mL or 2.2 mL of injectable solution in order for them to fit into different size syringes.

Checks before preparing local anaesthetics for patients

It is important to look at the patient's medical history to establish if there were any complications the last time he/she received a local anaesthetic. By undertaking this, the dental team can be prepared for any manifestation of an emergency.

PAIN AND ANXIETY CONTROL

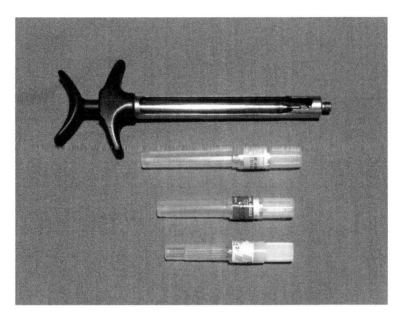

Figure 3.2 Sterile self-aspirating syringe and sterile disposable needle: gauges 27 (long), 30 and 31 (short and shorter).

The local anaesthetic syringe should be inspected to ensure that it is sterile and moves smoothly when pressed. The local anaesthetic cartridge itself should be checked to ensure the expiry date has not been reached, the solution is intact and not cloudy or discoloured, and the bungs have not been tampered with. The disposable needle to be assembled onto the self-aspirating syringe should be inspected to ensure it is the correct size for the type of injection being administered and that it is intact. The batch number and expiry date should be written in the patient's notes.

Types of local anaesthetic syringes

- **Self-aspirating syringe (Figure 3.1):** These are used to avoid the anaesthetic being injected into a blood vessel. If blood flowed into the cartridge, the clinician should stop the administration, reposition the needle and continue to inject the local anaesthetic solution into the chosen area until the blood disappeared.
- **Ligmaject/peripress (Figure 3.3):** This is a gun-shaped syringe that injects small amounts of anaesthetic under high pressure. A very short needle is used in conjunction with it to introduce/force the anaesthetic solution between the tooth and the bone into the periodontal ligaments.
- **Ultra-safety-plus disposable sterile syringe (Figure 3.4):** These sterile injectable systems are single-patient-use only. They have an integral protective sheath needlestick injury-prevention device.

PAIN AND ANXIETY CONTROL

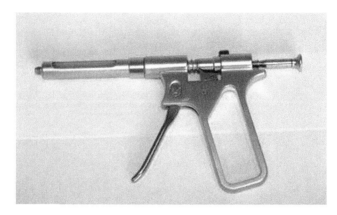

Figure 3.3 Ligmaject/peripress. Source: Hollins, C. 2013 *Levison's Textbook for Dental Nurses,* 11th edition, p. 394. Reproduced with permission of John Wiley & Sons.

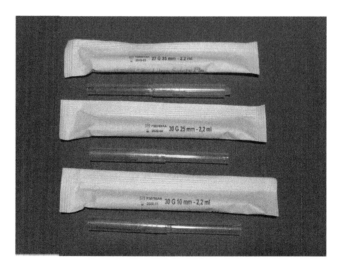

Figure 3.4 Ultra-safety-plus disposable sterile syringe.

Types of local anaesthetic

- Lignocaine (xylocaine) 2% and adrenaline 1 in 80,000. The half-life in the body is approximately 1.5–2 hours.
- Prilocaine (citanest) 3% and octopressin (felypressin) (Figure 3.1). The half-life of prilocaine is approximately 1–1.5 hours.
- Prilocaine 4% plain which is rapidly taken up into the system and will therefore not provide pain relief for long maxillofacial procedures or those where post-operative numbness will be beneficial.

- Articaine 4% solution with epinephrine 1:100,000 or 1:200,000. Articaine is also known as septocaine and is one of the most widely used local anaesthetic agents in many European countries. It has a half-life of approximately 20 minutes.

Typical contents of a local anaesthetic cartridge
- Anaesthetic agent.
- Vasoconstrictor.
- Reducing agent (sodium metabisulphate), which prevents oxidisation of the anaesthetic solution resulting in discolouration.
- Fungicide (thymol) which prevents clouding.
- Sterile water.

Complications that can occur during and after the administration of a local anaesthetic

When a local anaesthetic is administered complications can occur, such as:

- The patient could experience a medical emergency with the most common being a faint, especially when an inferior dental block has been given. This could be attributed to some of the local anaesthetic being accidently injected into a blood vessel, the patient being sat upright during the administration of the local anaesthetic, the patient feeling nervous, lack of food or too much clothing being worn.
- The needle could break during administration of a local anaesthetic.
- The patient could experience an allergic reaction to the local anaesthetic used.
- A blood vessel could be accidentally nicked and a haematoma or 'blood blister' could occur. This would eventually heal.
- If the needle is positioned too posteriorly during the administration of an inferior dental block (Figure 3.5), anaesthetic may penetrate the parotid gland causing transient facial paralysis. This would affect the facial nerve or the VIIth cranial nerve. As the patient will experience a temporary loss of their facial muscles, they would not be able to close their eyelid. If the needle is positioned too medially the medial pterygoid muscle can be injected, resulting in trismus (limited mouth opening).
- Nerve damage can occur during an injection. If this occurs the patient will experience paresthesia (numbness) which can take weeks or even months to return to normal; on occasions, the patient is left with permanent nerve damage.
- Following the procedure the patient could accidently self-inflict trauma by either biting their lip, tongue or sustaining a thermal burn caused by drinking hot fluids. This commonly occurs in children or those with learning difficulties.

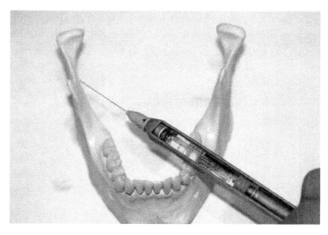

Figure 3.5 Inferior dental block technique. Source: Hollins, C. 2013 *Levison's Textbook for Dental Nurses*, 11th edition, p. 392. Reproduced with permission of John Wiley & Sons.

- The clinician or dental nurses could accidently sustain a needlestick injury. One could also occur by not following protocol when dealing with sharps.

  The following is therefore important:

- Correct local anaesthetic is administered to suit the patient's medical history.
- Careful placement of the needle during the administration.
- Care is taken while handling sharps (following guidelines/protocol).
- The patient fully understands the post-operative instructions.

Safe handling of needles

Following the administration of a local anaesthetic the needle will be contaminated; it must therefore be handled carefully to avoid injury to the dental team. They must always be placed in a rigid sealable container (Figure 3.6) that can be incinerated. Safety needles are available which have a plastic slide to protect the needle and allow it to be unscrewed from the syringe. In many organisations, the responsibility of dismantling the sharps lies with the clinician. The rationale for this is that they have already been exposed to risk by administration of the local anaesthetic.

Needlestick injury management

If a needlestick injury occurred the wound must be:

- Encouraged to bleed by holding it under running water.
- Dried and covered with a waterproof plaster or dressing.

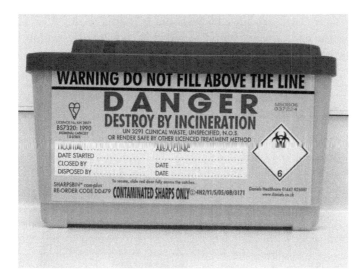

Figure 3.6 Sharps bin. Source: Rogers, N. 2011 *Basic Guide to Dental Sedation Nursing*, p. 35. Reproduced with permission of John Wiley & Sons.

It must not be:

- Scrubbed while washing it under running water.
- Sucked.

Once first aid attention has been administered, occupational health must be informed and an appointment made for further advice. If the needle has been used to treat a patient they would be requested to give a sample of blood.

Elimination of a local anaesthetic from the body

Local anaesthetic solutions are mainly metabolised by the liver, although they can also be broken down by the kidneys and the lungs.

Pre- and post-operative instructions

Patients should be advised that: they will feel a sharp scratch; it will take a few minutes to lose feeling in the area where the local anaesthetic has been administered; and the clinician will ensure the area is numb before starting any treatment. They should be told that the area may feel fatter than normal, but it isn't. Once treatment has been completed, they should be advised that it can take a few hours for the local anaesthetic to wear off and for full feeling to return. During this period they should be careful not to damage the area by avoiding eating on the affected side, not to have hot drinks and to be careful not to bite their cheek and lips. They should be told that the lip, if numb, will tingle when the area affected starts to return to normal. Depending upon the dental treatment received, they may be advised to take some painkillers if it is likely they will be in pain after the anaesthetic has worn off.

Types of injections

There are various types of injections (Figures 3.5 and 3.7) administered to patients undergoing maxillofacial surgery. The injection used will depend upon the treatment being received, the area within the mouth being anaesthetised and the associated nerve supply.

Infiltration

Infiltration injections are used when the dental treatment to be carried out is confined to one area within the mouth. The anaesthetic is administered over the apex of a tooth by placing the needle under the mucous membrane that covers the alveolar bone. This allows the anaesthetic to soak into the bone to reach the nerve endings of the tooth. Due to the action of this type of injection, it can only be administered in an area in the mouth where the compact bone is not only permeable but thin enough to allow the anaesthetic to enter the spongy bone. Infiltration injections are therefore administered to all the maxillary and the lower incisor teeth.

Nerve block

Nerve block injections are advantageous when an individual tooth has an infection present as the anaesthetic is administered away from the tooth, preventing

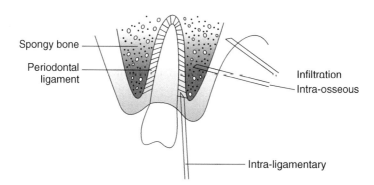

Figure 3.7 Types of injections. Source: Hollins, C. 2013 *Levison's Textbook for Dental Nurses*, 11th edition, p. 392. Reproduced with permission of John Wiley & Sons.

PAIN AND ANXIETY CONTROL

the infection from being spread. The most commonly used nerve block is the inferior dental block. This type of injection will produce anaesthesia of an entire area supplied by major trunks, so is therefore ideal when numerous teeth within that quadrant require anaesthetising. It works by the local anaesthetic being deposited into the nerve trunk as it passes through the soft tissues before entering the jaw, therefore preventing any painful sensations from reaching the brain. In the case of an inferior dental block the anaesthetic is deposited over the mandibular foramen. As the lingual nerve is in close proximity to the inferior dental nerve, it will also become anaesthetised. Other nerve block injections are the mental block and posterior superior nerve block.

Intraligamentary

An intraligamentary injection is where the local anaesthetic solution is forced into the periodontal ligament of a tooth. This type of injection is not commonly used on its own. It can be used when a nerve block injection has not been effective, thereby providing additional anaesthetic, or with an infiltration injection, as these combinations provide more profound anaesthesia. It cannot however be used if there is any gingival infection unless the tooth is to be extracted. A self-aspirating syringe cannot be used to administer this type of injection. A syringe that is tailor-made, such as a ligmaject (Figure 3.3) or citaject syringe, is required. These syringes have an integral plastic sheath that the 1.8 mL anaesthetic cartridge fits into, preventing any injuries should the cartridge break. The reason the cartridge could break is attributed to the force required to deposit the local anaesthetic solution, resulting in pressure building up. To counteract this pressure the syringe also has a ratchet-type plunger.

Intraosseous

An intraosseous injection (Figure 3.8) is where the anaesthetic is deposited directly into compact bone and into the spongy bone. The anaesthetic is placed adjacent to the tooth to be anaesthetised. A Stabident kit can be used, which comprises a contra-angled (slow speed) hand-piece-driven perforator, a solid 27-gauge wire with a bevelled end that, upon activation, drills a small hole into the cortical plate through which local anaesthetic solution can be administered, using a 27-gauge (ultra-short) needle. An intraosseous injection should not be used when there is gross periodontal disease present.

Injections administered for the upper and lower teeth

Prior to any maxillofacial surgery the patient receives the administration of local anaesthetic so that the treatment received is pain free. The type of injection

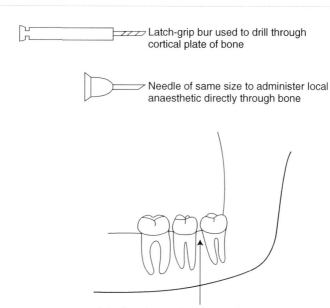

Latch-grip bur used to drill through cortical plate of bone

Needle of same size to administer local anaesthetic directly through bone

Injection site needs to be carefully chosen, between teeth and without damaging roots

Figure 3.8 Intraosseous system. Source: Hollins, C. 2013 *Levison's Textbook for Dental Nurses,* 11th edition, p. 394. Reproduced with permission of John Wiley & Sons.

administered will be decided by the maxillofacial surgeon. If extractions are planned, the type of injection is usually dependent upon the tooth or teeth to be extracted (Tables 3.1 and 3.2).

Table 3.1 Injections for the maxillary teeth

Tooth	Type of injection for extractions
1	Buccal and palatal infiltration
2	Buccal and palatal infiltration
3	Buccal and palatal infiltration
4	Buccal and palatal infiltration
5	Buccal and palatal infiltration
6	Buccal and palatal infiltration or superior dental block
7	Buccal and palatal infiltration or superior dental block
8	Buccal and palatal infiltration or superior dental block

Table 3.2 Injections for the mandibular teeth

Tooth	Type of injection for extractions
1	Inferior dental block or buccal infiltration
2	Inferior dental block or buccal infiltration
3	Inferior dental block
4	Inferior dental block
5	Inferior dental block
6	Inferior dental block and buccal infiltration
7	Inferior dental block and buccal infiltration
8	Inferior dental block and buccal infiltration

CONSCIOUS SEDATION

Patients may request, or be offered, a form of conscious sedation as an adjunct to help them accept dental treatment; some patients may be frightened or anxious in the dental environment, and treatment with local anaesthetic alone would not be tolerated.

Conscious sedation is defined as:

> … a technique in which the use of a drug or drugs produces a state of depression of the central nervous system, enabling treatment to be carried out, but during which verbal contact with the patient is maintained throughout the period of sedation. The drugs and techniques used to provide conscious sedation for dental treatment should carry a margin of safety wide enough to render loss of consciousness unlikely.
>
> Standards for Conscious Sedation in the Provision of Dental Care, 2015

Prior to patients being treated with conscious sedation, the clinician must establish the most appropriate form to provide. This will depend upon their knowledge and skills and that of their dental team along with the patient's medical, dental and social history so that safe sedation is provided. All emergency drugs and equipment must be available, with all staff being conversant with the management of medical emergencies. To achieve the aforementioned the patient should attend an assessment appointment where medical checks such as blood pressure and heart rate are performed, along with questions pertaining to any worries the patient may have. Their medical and social status will be discussed along with any treatment preferences. A dental examination will be carried out to formulate a treatment plan and consent is taken. The patient will be provided with pre- and post-operative instructions relating to the form of conscious sedation they are to receive together with an appointment. If the form of conscious sedation being requested by the patient or deemed the most appropriate by the clinician is not being offered or available at the dental practice being attended, patients may on occasions be referred to another specialist practice or the local general or dental hospital.

Intravenous sedation

What is intravenous sedation?

Intravenous sedation is when a drug, usually of the anti-anxiety variety, is administered into the blood system during dental treatment. The drug commonly administered is midazolam (Figure 3.9). The reason midazolam is commonly used is due to its action, whereby upon administration it rapidly results in a sedated patient with the patient recovering from its effects quickly. It has the ability to reduce patient anxieties and provide them with anterograde amnesia, which means not all patients will remember the dental treatment despite being aware at the time. However, it does have the disadvantage of requiring a cannula to be placed in order to administer the drug. This is usually a 22-gauge venflon (Figure 3.10). It can also minimally affect the cardiovascular system and can cause respiratory depression. Due to these disadvantages, the patient must be monitored carefully throughout their appointment by a second person, normally an appropriately trained dental nurse.

Patient monitoring

Monitoring a patient's vital signs commences as soon as they enter the dental surgery. Prior to the patient receiving treatment, the dental team should observe

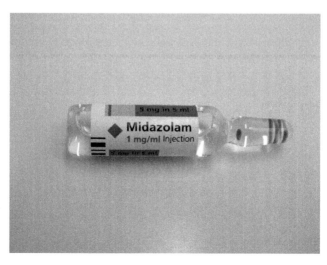

Figure 3.9 Ampoule of midazolam. Source: Rogers, N. 2011 *Basic Guide to Dental Sedation Nursing*, p. 71. Reproduced with permission of John Wiley & Sons.

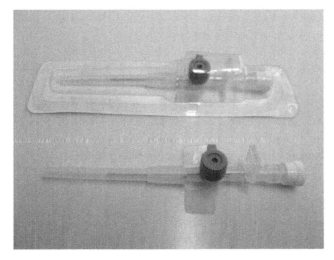

Figure 3.10 22-gauge venflon. Source: Rogers, N. 2011 *Basic Guide to Dental Sedation Nursing*, p. 27. Reproduced with permission of John Wiley & Sons.

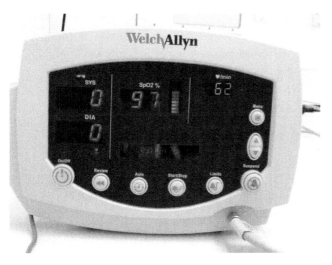

Figure 3.11 Pulse oximeter monitor. Source: Rogers, N. 2011 *Basic Guide to Dental Sedation Nursing*, p. 22. Reproduced with permission of John Wiley & Sons.

the patient's skin tone and demeanour. They will take the patient's blood pressure, respiratory rate and pulse. A pulse oximeter probe will be placed on the patient's finger to establish the amount of saturated oxygen attached to the haemoglobin. The use of a pulse oximeter is mandatory when patients receive intravenous sedation. However, it must not be relied upon as it is the clinical judgment of the dental team that is paramount; the pulse oximeter (Figure 3.11) can be affected by outside influences such as patient movement, cold hands, nail varnish and external lights. Monitoring will continue while dental treatment is undertaken, during the recovery phase of the patient's appointment and while they are being assessed for discharge.

For patients to be accepted for this form of sedation they must be able to comply with rigid pre- and post-operative instructions. The patient should:

- Bring an escort who can stay for the duration of the appointment and will chaperone the patient for the next 24 hours. The escort must be free of other responsibilities such as children or elderly relatives.
- Go home by car or taxi and not drive, operate any machinery or climb any ladders or scaffolding.
- Not make any important decisions or sign any legal documents.
- Take routine medication.
- Refrain from work for the next 24 hours.
- Not drink alcohol on the day of the appointment.
- Eat a light meal a few hours before their appointment.
- Clean their teeth prior to attending if having teeth removed.

Drugs used for intravenous sedation
Midazolam (hypnovel)
Midazolam is a schedule IV controlled substance which belongs to the family of drugs known as benzodiazepines. It is a clear odourless liquid in glass ampoules that can be obtained as:

- 10 mg in 5 mL.
- 10 mg in 2 mL.
- 5 mg in 5 mL.

To help prevent the risk of over-sedation, the recommended presentation for use in the dental surgery is 5 mg in 5 mL. Midazolam is a controlled drug and should therefore be under lock and key and treated as such. It produces sedation by acting on the central nervous system, reducing the excitability of neurones in the mid-brain. The dose provided to patients is dependent upon age but not weight, with it being slowly titrated over a period of time.

Flumazenil (annexate)
Flumazenil (Figure 3.12) is a schedule IV controlled substance which belongs to the family of drugs known as benzodiazepines. It is a clear liquid, obtained as 500 mcg in a 5 mL glass ampoule. It is the antidote for an overdose of a benzo-diazepine. It competitively inhibits the activity of the benzodiazepine, allowing the neurones to return to their normal state of excitability and reversing the sedative effect. Flumazenil is also a controlled drug and should be held in a secure location.

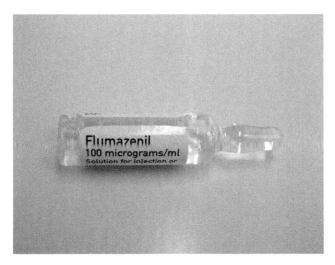

Figure 3.12 Ampoule of flumazenil. Source: Rogers, N. 2011 *Basic Guide to Dental Sedation Nursing*, p. 77. Reproduced with permission of John Wiley & Sons.

Inhalation sedation

Inhalation sedation is also known as relative analgesia. This form of conscious sedation has been described as 'representing the most nearly ideal clinical sedative circumstance'. It is commonly used for paediatric patients as it is non-invasive and does not require a cannula to be placed. This makes it ideal for the needle-phobic patient. It can be used in conjunction with intravenous sedation to allow cannulation to take place. Its onset is rapid, as is the patient's recovery with no post-operative restraints being placed on the patient. Patients may be offered an acclimatisation appointment where they are fitted for a mask (some clinicians permit their patients to take these home), shown the inhalation sedation machine (Figures 3.13 and 3.14) and allowed to briefly experience its effects.

What is inhalation sedation?
Inhalation sedation is the appropriate use of nitrous oxide combined with oxygen to produce a sedative/euphoric state. A patient sedates when nitrous oxide and oxygen are delivered through a nasal hood. Patients must be able to breathe through their nose and not have a cold, otherwise sedation will be ineffective. As the patient breathes the mixture of nitrous oxide and oxygen in, they travel through the respiratory system to reach the alveoli sacs within the lungs. It is here that the nitrous oxide diffuses across the membrane of the alveoli into the blood. It does this because one of the characteristics of gases is that they will transfer to another area if the concentration is lower than their current location.

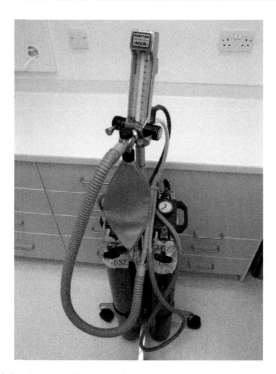

Figure 3.13 Mobile relative analgesia machine. Source: Rogers, N. 2011 *Basic Guide to Dental Sedation Nursing*, p. 83. Reproduced with permission of John Wiley & Sons.

The nitrous oxide then travels in the blood to the brain and within 3–5 minutes the patient will start to feel its effects. The continual provision of nitrous oxide maintains the sedated status until it is eliminated by switching the nitrous oxide off. Upon cessation of nitrous oxide, oxygen must be provided for 3–5 minutes at 100% to prevent the patient being left with a headache/hangover effect or not being able to breathe properly. Patients will not only sedate and feel relaxed, but will be provided with mild analgesia and some degree of anterograde amnesia.

Inhalation sedation machine

Inhalation sedation machines can either be mobile or piped systems. Whichever is used, they must be checked prior to the patient's appointment to ensure they are safe. This will involve carrying out a systematic check to ensure all the integral safety mechanisms are functional. For example, if the oxygen fails, the nitrous oxide will also cut off. All tubing will be inspected to make sure that there are no tears and a scavenging system will be attached. Scavenging systems are used to remove the waste nitrous oxide from the atmosphere so that it is not inhaled by the dental team.

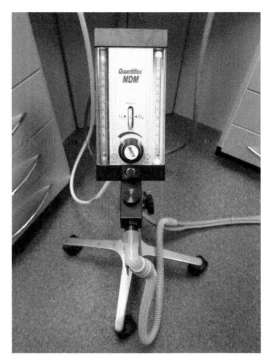

Figure 3.14 Piped relative analgesia machine. Source: Rogers, N. 2011 *Basic Guide to Dental Sedation Nursing*, p. 79. Reproduced with permission of John Wiley & Sons.

Patient monitoring

Patients must be monitored carefully throughout their appointment by a appropriately trained sedation nurse. Skin tone, breathing and demeanour are all important vital signs to monitor. The reservoir bag must be checked to ensure it is moving in and out to reflect the patient's chest movements and to ensure it is not over- or under-inflating. Clinicians do not always request any medical checks to be carried out at an assessment stage or on the day of the appointment. The use of a pulse oximeter is not mandatory; the inhalation sedation machine used will provide a minimum of 30% oxygen at all times, so the pulse oximeter will reflect this.

Transmucosal (off-licence) sedation

This form of conscious sedation is where the sedation drug is not being administered in the way for which it has been licensed and is therefore deemed an advanced technique. Midazolam is not licensed for oral use. However, there are lots of data available on its safety and efficacy when used orally by adding it to some cold tea or blackcurrant squash to mar its bitter taste for the patient to drink. Another route is intra nasal where a mucosal atomising device is used to squirt midazolam into the nose. Epistatus (buccal midazolam), the emergency drug for epilepsy, is also used for off-licence/transmucosal sedation. With any of these techniques the amount of midazolam used will be based on several factors such as the patient's age, physical health, history of drug use and anxiety levels. Some clinicians use one of these routes in conjunction with intravenous sedation and a cannula is placed. When this occurs the amount of midazolam will be reduced, taking into account the drug already received. What must be remembered when an off-licence sedation technique is used is that the drug being administered is the same as for intravenous sedation; it will therefore act upon the body in the same manner, resulting in the same effects. This means the rigid pre- and post-operative instructions that are mandatory for intravenous sedation also apply to off-licence/transmucosal sedation.

Patient monitoring

Monitoring a patient's vital signs commences as soon as they enter the dental surgery. Prior to the patient receiving treatment, the dental team should observe the patient's skin tone and demeanour. They will take the patient's blood pressure, respiratory rate and pulse. A pulse oximeter probe will be placed on the patient's finger to establish the amount of saturated oxygen attached to the haemoglobin. The use of a pulse oximeter is mandatory when patients receive off-licence/transmucosal sedation. It must not be relied upon however, as the clinical judgment of the dental team is paramount; the pulse oximeter can be affected by outside influences such as patient movement, cold hands, nail varnish and external lights. Monitoring will continue while dental treatment is undertaken, during the recovery phase of the patient's appointment and while they are being assessed for discharge.

Oral sedation and pre-mediaction

This is the lightest form of conscious sedation administered and is used to reduce a patient's anxiety levels prior to treatment. This form is universally accepted with patients being prescribed either an oral tablet or suspension which can be taken at a surgery (oral sedation) or at home (pre-medication). The dosage the patient receives depends upon their weight with temazepam being the drug commonly prescribed. Temazepam belongs to the same family of drugs as midazolam used for intravenous sedation (benzodiazepines), meaning patients must comply with the same pre- and post-operative instructions. Some clinicians use a form of oral sedation in conjunction with intravenous sedation and place a cannula. When this occurs the amount of midazolam will be reduced, taking into account the drug already received.

Patient monitoring

A patient's vital signs should be monitored in the same way as for intravenous and transmucosal (off-licence) sedation as described above.

GENERAL ANAESTHETIC

General anaesthesia must only be carried out in a hospital setting that has suitable critical care facilities. It is a state of controlled sleep (medically induced coma) where a patient is rendered unconscious through the administration of a combination of drugs that stop the messages from the nerves in the body being recognised by the brain. This means that they will not feel any pain or sensations, nor will they remember the procedure. As the anaesthetic wears off the patient will regain consciousness. An anaesthetist administers the anaesthetic either through a cannula or they may ask the patient to breathe in the anaesthetic gases and oxygen via a mask controlled by an anaesthetic machine. The patient may have a tube inserted into the mouth to help them breathe during the procedure. The anaesthetist stays for the duration of the procedure to monitor the patient's heart rate, blood pressure and the amount of oxygen in their blood by interpreting the machines to which the patient is connected. These machines monitor the activity of the heart and other body systems. The anaesthetist may also provide the patient with other drugs during the procedure.

When maxillofacial surgery is undertaken, a local anaesthetic is administered to provide post-operative pain relief for the patient. In addition, the effects of the vasoconstrictor will reduce bleeding. This is beneficial as it will help to provide a clear field of vision for the clinician.

Before a patient receives a general anaesthetic they must attend a pre-operative assessment. At this appointment the patient is assessed to ensure they are fit for the procedure. This involves the taking and recording of their medical history and blood pressure, pulse and respiratory rate. At this appointment the patient has the procedure explained to them with written consent being obtained. The patient is advised of the pre- and post-operative instructions that they must comply with:

- No food or drink should be consumed for 6 hours prior to appointment.
- If they have a cold, cough, or sore throat, to contact the hospital.
- To take their normal medication on the day of their appointment unless advised not to by the anaesthetist.
- Patients should be accompanied by a responsible adult. A child must be with a parent or legal guardian.
- To wear loose clothing.
- Remove all jewellery, nail varnish, artificial teeth or removable orthodontic appliances.

PAIN AND ANXIETY CONTROL

- To visit the toilet before the procedure.
- Not to drive, operate any machinery, sign legal documents or drink alcohol for the next 24 hours.
- To arrange for someone to drive him/her home and stay with them for the next 24 hours.
- To have pain relief at home that is normally taken for a headache, but not aspirin.

On the day of the general anaesthetic the patient will be asked various questions relating to their medical history, how they are feeling and whether they have complied with the pre-operative instructions. This is undertaken to ensure that the procedure runs smoothly without any complications.

Once the procedure is completed, the patient is moved into a recovery room where they will still be attached to the monitors and provided with oxygen. Once the anaesthetist and recovery nurse are happy with the progress of the patient, the monitors will be disconnected. Depending upon the maxillofacial surgery undertaken and whether the patient is a day case or not, they will either be discharged into the care of their escort or taken back to the ward. If the patient is a day case the cannula will be removed, they will be offered something to eat and drink and provided with post-operative instructions. During the recovery phase patients can shiver, feel sick, disorientated and sleepy, and may complain of a sore throat.

PAIN AND ANXIETY CONTROL

Chapter 4

Assessment clinics, equipment and medicaments used during complex procedures

LEARNING OUTCOMES

At the end of this chapter you should have an understanding of:

1. The role of the dental nurse during patient assessment clinics.
2. The equipment and medicaments used during complex procedures.

INTRODUCTION

Within a maxillofacial and oral surgery department different clincs can run parallel with one another. They are catergorised as being either an assessment or treatment clinic. Assessment clinics involve the patient being assessed by a maxillofacial surgeon. Once assessed the patient is either listed for a procedure for further investigations, kept under consultant review, given advice or a prescription, or discharged back to the referring dentist or doctor's care. Treatment clinics, as the name suggests, involve the patient undergoing a type of treatment or procedure. These patients have already been assessed by a maxillofacial consultant or a clinician within the maxillofacial team. They have previously been listed for the planned procedure to either treat or ameliorate a diagnosed condition. If a biopsy was listed, this will aid the maxillofacial consultant or clinician in gaining a definitive diagnosis. In either case, the basic role of the dental nurse involves the same responsibilities and skills required whenever a patient receives dental treatment.

Basic Guide to Oral and Maxillofacial Surgery, First Edition. Nicola Rogers and Cinzia Pickett.
© 2017 John Wiley & Sons Ltd. Published 2017 by John Wiley & Sons Ltd.

Prior to the clinic commencing, the dental nurse assigned to the clinic should undertake a pre-clinic check. The dental nurse should ensure that any previously ordered images or reports for patients attending a review appointment are available for the consultant. The consultation room is made ready by undertaking cross-infection control procedures and preparing any items that may be required during the consultation. The session list should be checked for any new referrals, along with establishing if any relevant radiographs are attached to the referral and, if so, these are available for the clinician. If none are provided by the referring clinican and there is a possibility that an image may be required, this should be highlighted to the clinician so that a request for one can be made.

An assessment appointment comprises several different elements. These may include:

- Greeting the patient.
- Recording the patient's height, weight and body mass index (BMI).
- Clinician recording the patient's medical, social and dental history.
- Discussion regarding the reason for referral.
- Clinical examination.
- Radiographic examination.
- Patient's pathway discussed in respect of further investigations and, dependent upon outcome, possible treatment plans.
- Consent may be taken.
- Advice provided.
- Patient discharged and return to referrer's care.

ASSESSMENT CLINICS, EQUIPMENT AND MEDICAMENTS

EQUIPMENT AND MEDICAMENTS USED DURING COMPLEX PROCEDURES

Drills, burs and irrigation

During surgical procedures bone removal may be necessary to expose underlying teeth and structures. To undertake this, a surgical hand-piece (Figure 4.1) with long flexible irrigation tubing attached is used. The solution used for irrigation is 0.9% sodium chloride. This comes in large bags which are single-use. A surgical hand-piece will have an intergral thin metal tube that one end of the irrigation tubing is connected to. The other end is attached to a surgical hand-piece motorised unit that passes the sodium chloride through the tubing when the hand-piece is in use. If this system is not available, the dental nurse will be requested to irrigate using a sterile disposable syringe (Figure 4.2) 0.9% containing sodium chloride (Figure 4.3) to avoid the bur

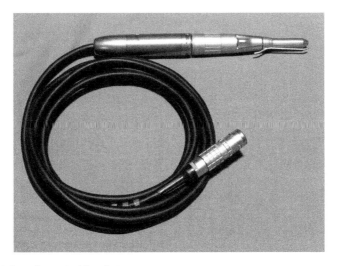

Figure 4.1 Straight surgical hand-piece.

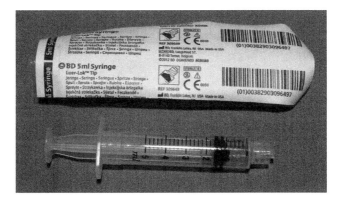

Figure 4.2 5 mL sterile disposable syringe.

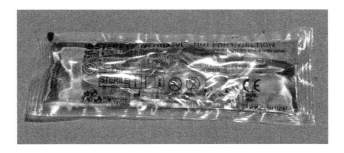

Figure 4.3 0.9% sodium chloride sachet.

ASSESSMENT CLINICS, EQUIPMENT AND MEDICAMENTS

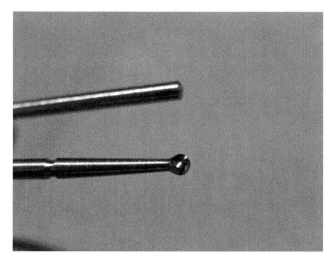

Figure 4.4 No. 6 rosehead surgical bur.

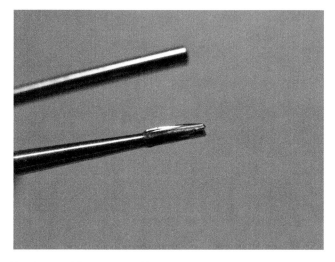

Figure 4.5 No. 4 tapered fissure surgical bur.

overheating and aid the clinican's vision. The commonly used surgical burs are a No. 6 rosehead (Figure 4.4) and No. 4 tapered or flat fissured bur (Figure 4.5). The rosehead bur is used to remove bone and the flat fissured bur to bisect a tooth for easier removal.

Blades

A surgical scalpel is formed of two components: the handle and the blade. These components can either be: separate, where the blade is disposed of after

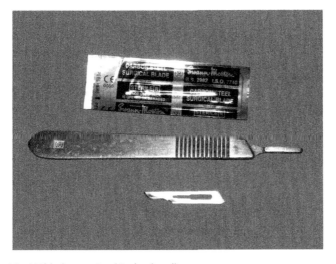

Figure 4.6 No. 15 blade on a Bard-Parker handle.

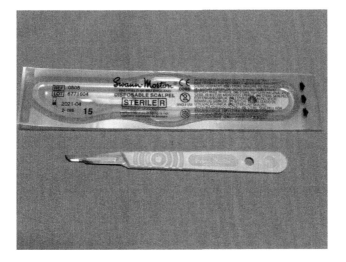

Figure 4.7 Disposable No. 15 scalpel blade and handle.

ASSESSMENT CLINICS, EQUIPMENT
AND MEDICAMENTS

use and the handle decontaminated and sterilised; or combined into one unit, when both the handle and blade are disposed of after use to reduce the risk of a sharps injury. The blade size frequently used in maxillofacial surgery is a No. 15 (Figures 4.6 and 4.7). This blade has a small, curved cutting edge and is ideal for making small, short, precise incisions. It can be used intra-orally when performing procedures such as biopsies and also extra-orally on skin procedures. A No. 11 blade has a pointed end used for incison and drainage (Figure 4.8).

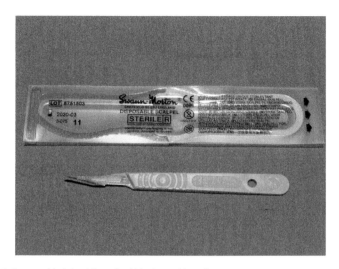

Figure 4.8 Disposable No. 11 scalpel blade and handle.

Disposal of blades

When dealing with sharps great care needs to be demonstrated. The clinician is responsible for maintaining the safety of the sharps and also for their safe disposal. If a separate scalpel system is in use then the clinician may wish to use a blade removal system; however, some clinicians prefer to use the Kilner needle holders to remove the blade. In either case the blade needs to be placed directly into the sharps container.

Sutures

Sutures are categorised as being either absorbable, non-absorbable, monofilament or braided. Each type has specific site usage, these being dependent on the advantages and disadvantages of the thread material. The number on the packaging (e.g. 3-0) determines the gauge of the thread.

Absorbable sutures

Vicryl Rapide™ (Polyglactin 910) is a synthetic, absorbable, braided sterile suture. Used for short-term wound closure, it is commonly used in outpatients for closure after procedures such as extractions (3-0) and biopsies (4-0), and also for subcutaneous muscle and fat when closing facial lacerations. As a braided suture it provides a good level of strength and knot security (Figure 4.9).

Monocryl™ (Poliglecaprone 25) is a synthetic, absorbable, monofilament sterile suture. As a monofilament suture it produces less tissue drag. The absorption of this suture is prolonged; at full absorption is takes longer than that of Polyglactin 910 sutures (Figure 4.10).

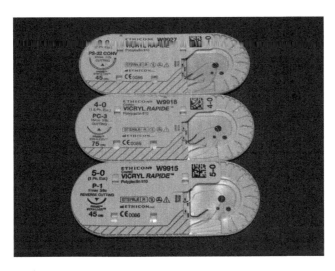

Figure 4.9 Vicryl sutures.

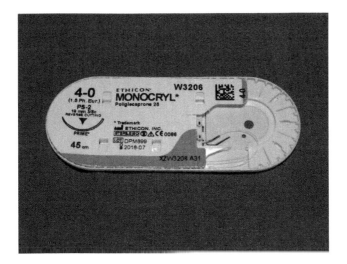

Figure 4.10 Monocryl suture.

Non-absorbable sutures

Novafill™ is a monofilament, polybutester, non-absorbable sterile suture. As a monofilament it produces less tissue drag and causes minimal inflammatory response, and as a polybutester it maintains its strength during healing. In maxillofacial scenarios it is commonly used on facial wounds as a 5-0 or 6-0 (Figure 4.11).

Sofsilk™ is a silk, non-absorbable, braided sterile suture. It uses include soft tissue, neuro and ophthalmic surgery and also for ligation (Figure 4.12).

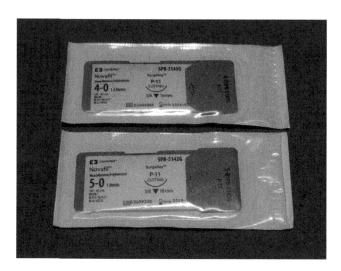

Figure 4.11 Novafil sutures.

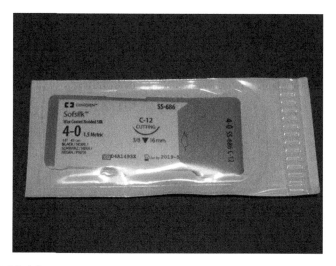

Figure 4.12 Sofsilk suture.

ASSESSMENT CLINICS, EQUIPMENT AND MEDICAMENTS

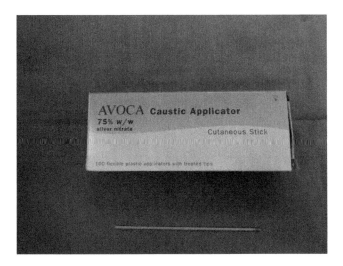

Figure 4.13 Silver nitrate.

Non-absorabable sutures require that the patient attend another appointment for suture removal.

Haemostatic agents

This group of topical agents work by promoting haemostasis; the formation of a blood clot to arrest bleeding. Silver nitrate (Figure 4.13) is an effective haemostat when suturing an area is difficult, such as after a biopsy on the palate. The silver nitrate is applied as the tip of a manufactured applicator. Once the tip has been moistened by either body fluid or water, the silver nitrate penetrates and is absorbed by the epidermal layer. After successful application, the area will have a black stained appearance and the patient should be reassured that this colouration is temporary and expected.

Absorbable haemostatic agents such as oxidised regenerated cellulose (Surgicel®; Figure 4.14) aid the patient's natural clotting process and are particularly useful when performing extractions on a warfarinised or medically compromised patient. It presents as a woven fabric mesh which is cut to size and placed with either college tweezers or Spencer Wells artery forceps, where the fabric absorbs blood forming a glutinous dark brown mass. Should it be indicated, the clinician may also wish to place sutures to aid closure and prevent the haemostatic agent from being lost.

Alvogel

Alvogel (Figure 4.15) is an antiseptic and analgesic. It is used as a local treatment for dry sockets (alveolar osteitis). It contains butamben, eugenol and

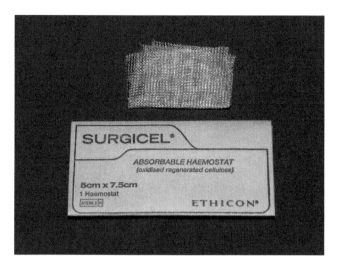

Figure 4.14 Surgicel.

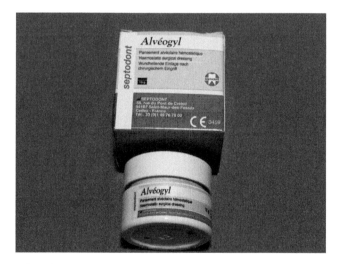

Figure 4.15 Alvogel.

idoform in the form of a fibrous brown paste. When a patient presents with a dry socket, the dentist will place it into the socket with college tweezers following irrigation.

Suction unit

Surgical suction units are required to remove fluids, predominately water and blood, produced during surgical procedures. This aids visibility for the clinician

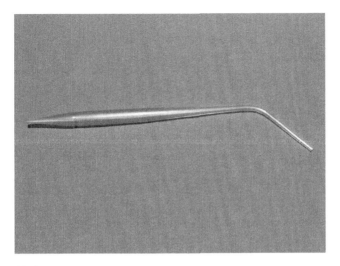

Figure 4.16 Yankaeur suction tip.

and also patient comfort. The unit is normally a trolley style to allow ease of positioning. Sterile tubing and suction tip (Figure 4.16) are attached to the unit and a clear, disposable container collects the fluid. If the unit is within the patient's sight, a drape may be placed over the container to prevent any patient anxiety over the amount of fluid being collected.

Diathermy

A diathermy machine when used will either coagulate or cut the soft tissue it is being used upon. An electrical current passes through a fine metal tip. When used for maxillofacial surgical procedures, the term electrosurgery is commonly used. Types of procedures that a diathermy machine might be used for are as follows:

- Sealing severed blood vessels by cauterisation.
- Cutting small areas of tissue, for example canine exposure.
- Removal of the operculum that lies over a partially erupted wisdom tooth.

There are two types of diathermy used in maxillofacial surgery: monopolar and bipolar. Monopolar is when the electrical current passes through the tip and through the patient. In this situation, the patient must sit on either a pad or hold a special rod. Bipolar is where the electrical current passes through one side of the tip and back up the other. As bipolar does not send a flow of electricity through the patient, its use is appropriate for carrying out microsurgery and for use with patients who have cardiac pacemakers fitted. As a diathermy machine generates heat, the maxillofacial team must be careful to avoid burning the patient during its use.

Cryosurgery

Cryosurgery is used to destroy abnormal or diseased tissue by the application of extreme cold to achieve an inflammatory and/or destructive response. As the mouth is smooth and humid, it provides an ideal environment for this technique. When cryosurgery is performed in the mouth very good results are achieved.

Cryosurgery works by freezing the cells; when their temperature drops to a specific point, ice crystals form inside to break them up. Further damage occurs once the blood vessels supplying the affected tissue begin to freeze. The frequently used solution for freezing lesions is liquid nitrogen as it is very cold.

It can be applied to diseased tissue using the probe of a cryojet, which is the most common method, sprayed on or patted on using a swab. When a cryojet is used liquid nitrogen is placed into it leaving an approximately 5 cm gap at the top. When the lid of the cryojet is placed, the liquid nitrogen becomes pressurised and freezes the probe that is attached to the flask. The lesion is covered with KY jelly or Vaseline and the probe placed upon it to allow the freezing process to take place. Once freezing is complete, the probe is removed.

Successful cell destruction varies with the speed and frequency of the thaw–freeze cycle. The rate of freezing must be rapid and the rate of thawing must be slow and unassisted. Upon successful treatment, the lesion becomes swollen (oedematous) and red (erythematous) and can ooze fluid. After 24 hours the area becomes dark, and within a few days a scab will form which can take several weeks to shed. The risk of using cryosurgery is that the adjacent healthy tissues can be damaged.

Chapter 5

Extractions

REASONS FOR EXTRACTIONS

Exodontia, commonly known as a dental extraction, is where a tooth or its roots are removed from its socket within the alveolar ridge. The tooth being removed could be a deciduous or a permanent tooth. Most dental practices undertake the removal of straightforward extractions on a daily basis using a local anaesthetic to provide pain-free treatment. Some patients will not tolerate a tooth being removed with a local anaesthetic only. In this instance the clinician will either refer the patient to another specialist dental surgery or local hospital where the patient can receive either a form of conscious sedation or a general anaesthetic. Naturally, if the dental surgery provides conscious sedation in house the patient may be treated within. Patients have teeth extracted for various reasons:

- **Pain:** to relieve the patient of pain.
- **Alveolar abscess:** to remove the infection to prevent a recurrence.

Basic Guide to Oral and Maxillofacial Surgery, First Edition. Nicola Rogers and Cinzia Pickett.
© 2017 John Wiley & Sons Ltd. Published 2017 by John Wiley & Sons Ltd.

- **Caries:** the tooth is un-restorable.
- **Impaction:** the patient has experienced several episodes of pericoronitis (infection) attributed to food packing in this area due to a partially erupted or impacted tooth.
- **Failed root canal therapy:** several attempts have been undertaken to root fill the tooth but have failed.
- **Orthodontics:** to allow the remaining teeth to be aligned or retracted.
- **Orthognathic:** the wisdom teeth are removed prior to the pre-surgical orthodontic stage.
- **Periodontal disease:** the tooth/teeth have become mobile due to the supporting structures of the teeth being destroyed.
- **Prosthetics:** if a patient has a tooth which isn't stable that may hinder the wearing of a partial denture, the tooth may be extracted.
- **Cosmetic:** if a tooth or teeth are not aesthetically pleasing then patients may choose to have them extracted so that they can be replaced with a bridge, denture or implant depending upon specific factors.
- **Patient choice:** the patient may not be able to afford the cost of restorative treatment or may not be able, or want to, commit to the number of appointments that would be necessary for restorative work to be carried out.
- **Supernumerary teeth:** where there is associated pathology present, a supernumerary tooth could delay tooth eruption or during orthodontic treatment it could increase the risk of caries occurring.
- **Deciduous teeth:** these may be extracted to allow their permanent replacements to erupt.

PRE- AND POST-OPERATIVE INSTRUCTIONS

Verbal and written pre- and post-operative care instructions are provided to patients to avoid any unnecessary complications. Pre-operative instructions comprise the following:

- Clean teeth prior to attending, as a clean mouth will heal more quickly.
- Have a light snack a few hours before their appointment to avoid any complications such as a faint.
- Take routine medications unless otherwise advised by the clinician to avoid their medical condition manifesting in the dental surgery.
- Bring any reliever medications that they may require for their medical condition (e.g. an inhaler for asthma).
- Bring someone with them for support.
- Bring a portable music system if they wish to, such as an iPod.
- Take the rest of the day off from school or work so that they can rest.
- Have some pain relief at home that is normally taken for a headache, but not aspirin as this is an anti coagulant (blood thinning agent).

EXTRACTIONS

Patients should also be advised that they will receive an appropriate amount of local anaesthetic to have the tooth removed, which will provide them with pain relief.

Post-operative instructions include:

- Avoid poking the socket with their tongue or fingers or bite their cheeks and lips, as this will result in trauma.
- Avoid eating soft or spicy foods or those which could easily become trapped within the socket.
- Avoid rinsing their mouths out for 24 hours to avoid clot disturbance.
- Have hot salt mouth washes (HSMW) after every meal for at least a week to keep the socket clean and promote healing. To make a HSMW, the patient should add a teaspoon of salt to comfortably hot water.
- Rest when at home, but to avoid taking a hot bath or sitting by a fire or in an over-heated room.
- Refrain from exercise or drinking alcohol or hot drinks for at least 24 hours after the procedure, as this will raise the blood pressure resulting in clot disturbance and possible haemorrhage.
- Refrain from smoking for as long as possible to prevent a dry socket occurring.
- If bleeding occurs, to roll up the swab provided and bite down hard for 20 minutes. If the bleeding persists, contact the dental surgery.

Coupled with the above instructions, patients should be advised that they will feel numb for a few hours after the procedure and may experience some pain, bruising and swelling following the extraction.

STRAIGHTFORWARD EXTRACTION

Procedure

Prior to a straightforward or simple extraction taking place, the maxillofacial surgeon must take the appropriate X-ray to aid diagnosis and treatment planning. They will then discuss the options with the patient in order for them to give consent. Once consent has been taken, the patient may or may not have the tooth extracted that day. If the patient is asked to attend another appointment for the extraction to be undertaken, they will be provided with pre-operative verbal and written instructions. If the patient has the tooth extracted during that appointment, they are provided with post-operative care instructions.

On the day of the extraction consent will be checked, along with ensuring that the correct patient is present. The patient's medical history is re-checked and any changes noted. Personal protective equipment will be placed on the patient and a brief explanation of the procedure provided. For pain and anxiety control the clinician may apply a topical anaesthetic prior to administering the

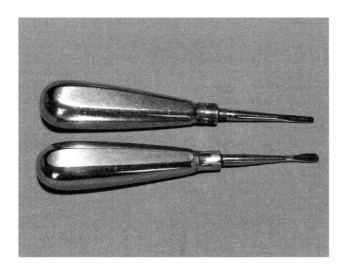

Figure 5.1 A luxator.

local anaesthetic. The patient is constantly monitored and reassured. The area surrounding the tooth to be extracted is checked to ensure that it is numb.

Once the maxillofacial surgeon is happy that the local anaesthetic is active, they will use either a luxator (Figure 5.1) or Coupland's chisel (Figure 5.2) to break the periodontal ligaments to detach them from the alveolar bone. Once this is completed, the maxillofacial surgeon will use the appropriate dental extraction forceps to remove the tooth/teeth. The patient will be advised that there will be some pushing, wiggling and pulling taking place.

Once the tooth has been removed, it will be inspected to ensure all the roots are intact and a rolled-up sterile swab (Figure 5.3) placed in the socket area. The patient will be asked to bite down on the swab for 15–20 minutes to allow haemostasis to take place. During this time the verbal and written post-operative care instructions are provided. Once haemostasis has been achieved, the patient is discharged and provided with further appointments if necessary.

Role of dental nurse

The dental nurse will prepare the dental surgery prior to the patient's arrival. They will carry out comprehensive infection control by disinfecting the primary and secondary zones and ensure that all instruments required for the planned extraction(s) selected are sterile. They will collect the patient's notes or ensure they are ready on the computer and display the radiographs. They will note the patient's medical history to establish if there are any special requirements for the patient, checking that consent has been taken.

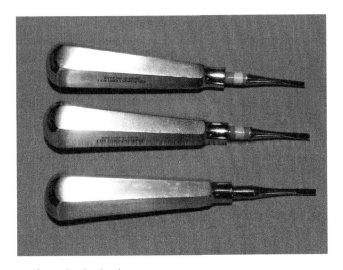

Figure 5.2 Set of Coupland's chisels.

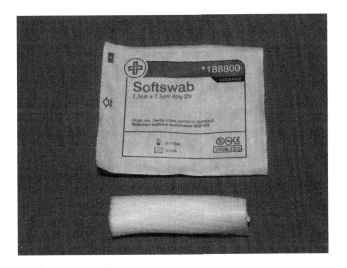

Figure 5.3 Rolled-up sterile swab.

The dental nurse will collect the patient from the waiting room, checking that they have the correct patient and introduce themselves. They will ask him/her if they have eaten and adhered to the pre-operative instructions provided at the last appointment and if they have any medication they would like placed on the work-surface. They will take the patient's coat and belongings and ask them to take a seat in the dental chair.

Once the patient is settled they will apply the personal protective equipment in the form of a bib and glasses, explaining to the patient the rationale for each. During the placement of the local anaesthetic, which the dental nurse will hand to the maxillofacial surgeon, they will monitor and reassure the patient, looking for signs of distress.

When the tooth is being removed the dental nurse may be requested to support the patient's head to keep it still. They may also need to provide some aspiration to remove the blood and saliva, providing a clear field of vision for the clinician as well as making it more comfortable for the patient. They will pass the elevators and extraction forceps as they are required and wipe them clean after each use to prevent the congealing of blood and debris.

Finally, once the tooth has been removed they will provide a rolled-up sterile swab which will be placed in the socket to achieve haemostasis. Throughout the procedure they will constantly monitor and reassure the patient, praising them. They will also ensure excellent cross-infection control and the health and safety of all. If requested, the dental nurse may provide verbal and written post-operative care instructions. Once the patient has left they will dispose of the waste correctly and carry out infection control procedures in the form of disinfection and sterilisation, returning the patient's notes and radiographs to file.

Forceps used

The maxillofacial surgeon will use forceps designed to extract specific teeth. Forceps used for the lower teeth are angulated at a right angle whereas forceps used for upper teeth are not, making them easily identifiable for the dental nurse.

Upper extraction forceps: permanent teeth

Upper straight permanent anterior extraction forceps (Figure 5.4) are designed to extract the upper right and upper left:

- Incisor teeth.
- Canine teeth.
- Retained roots.

Upper permanent pre-molar extraction forceps (Figure 5.5) are designed to extract the upper right and upper left:

- First and second pre-molar teeth.
- Retained roots.
- Third molar tooth.

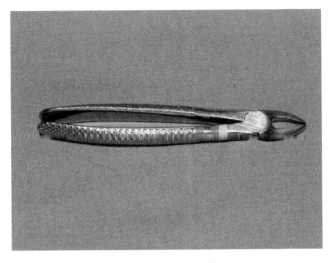

Figure 5.4 Upper straight permanent anterior extraction forceps.

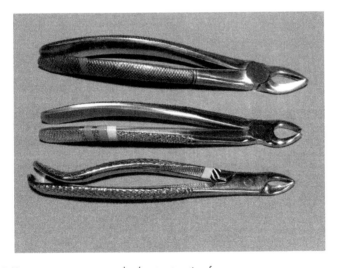

Figure 5.5 Upper permanent pre-molar/root extraction forceps.

Upper permanent molar extraction forceps (Figure 5.6) are designed to extract the upper right and left:

- First molar tooth.
- Second molar tooth.
- Third molar tooth.

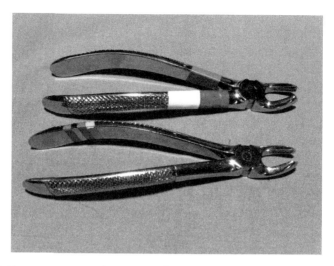

Figure 5.6 Upper permanent molar extraction forceps.

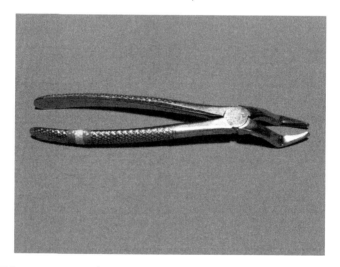

Figure 5.7 Bayonet extraction forceps.

Bayonet extraction forceps (Figure 5.7) are designed to extract the upper right and left:

- Third molar tooth.

Upper permanent eagle beak extraction forceps (Figure 5.8) are designed to extract the upper and left:

- First molar tooth.
- Second molar tooth.
- Third molar tooth.

EXTRACTIONS

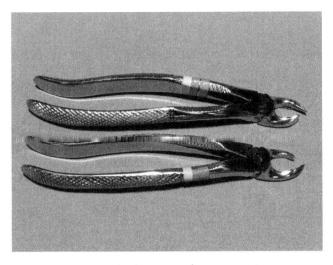

Figure 5.8 Upper permanent eagle beak extraction forceps.

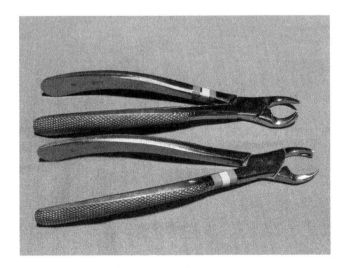

Figure 5.9 Upper permanent cowhorn extraction forceps.

Upper permanent cowhorn extraction forceps (Figure 5.9) are designed to extract the upper right and upper left:

- First molar tooth.
- Second molar tooth.
- Third molar tooth.

Upper supernumerary extraction forceps (Figure 5.10) are designed to extract extra teeth such as palatal canines.

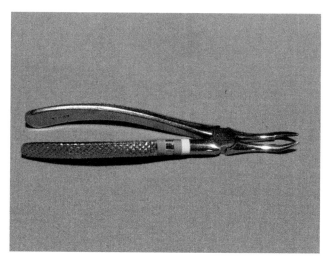

Figure 5.10 Upper supernumerary extraction forceps.

Upper permanent molar extraction, eagle beak and cowhorn forceps all have a left and right; the principle used when selecting these forceps is that the beak of the blade of the forceps is placed towards the cheek.

Lower extraction forceps: permanent teeth

Lower permanent root extraction forceps (Figure 5.11) are designed to extract the lower right and left:

- Incisor teeth.
- Canine teeth.
- First and second pre-molar teeth.

Lower permanent molar extraction forceps (Figure 5.12) are designed to extract the lower right and left:

- First molar tooth.
- Second molar tooth.
- Third molar tooth.

Lower permanent eagle beak extraction forceps (Figure 5.13) are designed to extract the lower right and left:

- First molar tooth.
- Second molar tooth.
- Third molar tooth.

EXTRACTIONS

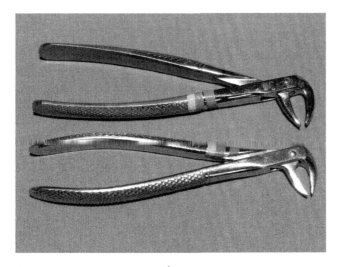

Figure 5.11 Lower permanent root extraction forceps.

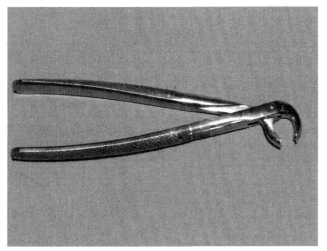

Figure 5.12 Lower permanent molar extraction forceps.

Lower permanent cowhorn extraction forceps (Figure 5.14) are designed to extract the lower right and left:

- First molar tooth.
- Second molar tooth.
- Third molar tooth.

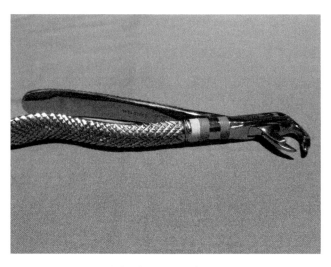

Figure 5.13 Lower permanent eagle beak extraction forceps.

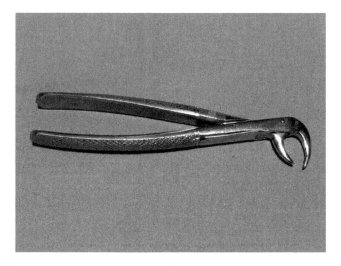

Figure 5.14 Lower permanent cowhorn extraction forceps.

Upper extraction forceps: deciduous teeth

Upper straight deciduous anterior extraction forceps (Figure 5.15) are designed to extract the upper right and upper left:

- Incisor teeth.
- Canine teeth.

Upper root deciduous extraction forceps (Figure 5.16) are designed to extract the upper right and left first molar tooth and retained roots.

EXTRACTIONS

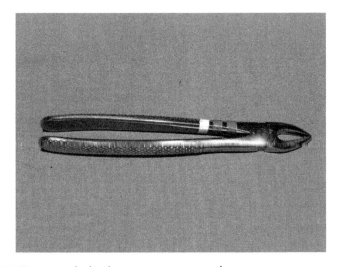

Figure 5.15 Upper straight deciduous anterior extraction forceps.

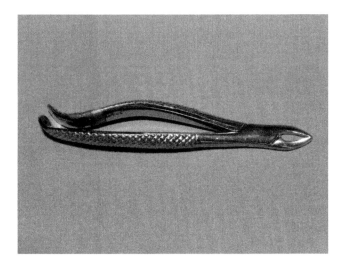

Figure 5.16 Upper root deciduous extraction forceps.

Upper molar deciduous extraction forceps (Figure 5.17) are designed to extract the upper left and right second molar tooth. Unlike the permanent molar extraction forceps, the deciduous molar extraction forceps will remove both the left and the right second molar teeth.

Lower extraction forceps: deciduous teeth

Lower root deciduous extraction forceps (Figure 5.18) are designed to extract the lower left and right:

EXTRACTIONS

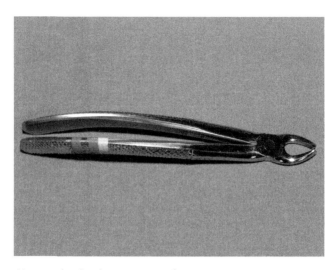

Figure 5.17 Upper molar deciduous extraction forceps.

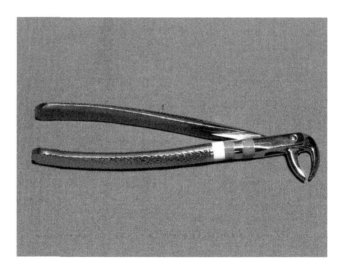

Figure 5.18 Lower root deciduous extraction forceps.

- Incisor teeth.
- Canine teeth.
- First molar teeth.
- Retained roots.

Lower molar deciduous extraction forceps (Figure 5.19) are designed to extract the lower left and right second molar tooth.

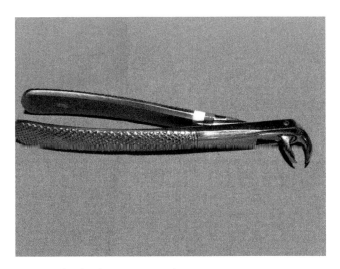

Figure 5.19 Lower molar deciduous extraction forceps.

EXTRACTIONS WITH COMPLICATIONS

Not all extractions are straightforward, even if it is perceived that they will be. Complications can occur, as described in the following sections.

Haemorrhage (bleeding)

There are three types of haemorrhage referred to when maxillofacial procedures are undertaken. These are primary, reactionary and secondary.

- **Primary** is perfectly normal, occurring at the time of surgery and should arrest within 4–8 minutes. Further haemorrhaging is avoided by the patient biting down on a sterile swab following an extraction. The maxillofacial surgeon should ensure haemostasis has been achieved prior to the patient being discharged, and that the patient has received the post-operative instructions which are provided verbally and in written format.
- **Reactionary** haemorrhage may follow primary haemorrhage, occurring a few hours later (usually 4–6 hours). This type of haemorrhage is a failure of coagulation. This may be because of the vasoconstrictor in the local anaesthetic wearing off, anticoagulant medications; or the patient not adhering to the care/advice provided, resulting in the loss of the blood clot. In this case the patient should bite down on the sterile swab provided for 20 minutes. If in that time the haemorrhaging does not arrest, the patient should contact the maxillofacial team. The patient should be reassured that this can be resolved and advised that blood mixed with saliva looks worse than it is. The

patient would be told to return so that the socket site can be inspected. Upon arrival, the patient would be provided with further reassurance and personal protective equipment. They would be instructed to bite down on another sterile swab. The maxillofacial surgeon would, if needed, place an absorbable haemostatic agent such as oxidised regenerated cellulose (Surgicel®; Figure 4.14) in the socket. If necessary the Surgicel® will be sutured in place, requiring administration of a local anaesthetic. Before discharge, the post-operative care instructions would be reiterated.

- **Secondary** haemorrhage occurs after 24 hours and can be attributed to an infection, possibly caused by a dirty mouth, stagnating food, pus entering the bloodstream from an abscess that was present and re-infecting the socket, or un-sterile items and fingers being placed in the mouth. The treatment is the same as for a reactionary haemorrhage, except that the maxillofacial surgeon may irrigate the socket site.

Dry socket (alveolar osteitis)

This condition occurs due to the loss of a blood clot which results in inflammation of the alveolar bone. Dry sockets are more common in posterior teeth than in anterior teeth, with the most common site being the third mandibular molar. Dry sockets are more common in the mandible than they are in the maxilla due to the nature of the bone in the mandible being more dense, the fact that food debris can be trapped more easily and the somewhat lower blood supply.

The causes of a dry socket are difficult extractions where the blood vessels are crushed, resulting in the inability of a clot to form. Secondary factors can be smoking, early or excessive mouth rinsing or the presence of an existing infection leading to bacteria re-entering the socket site and preventing a blood clot from forming.

The signs and symptoms of a dry socket are: slight swelling and redness around the soft tissues surrounding the socket site; exposed bone may be visible; the socket may be full of food debris or void of anything; sensitive to touch; a dull aching throb in that area which can radiate to other parts of the head; and halitosis or an unpleasant taste in the mouth.

Treatment of a dry socket would be analgesics for the pain, irrigation of the socket with either 0.9% sodium chloride (Figure 4.3) or chlorhexidine and the placement of alvogel (Figure 4.15) which will naturally abrade, and reiteration of the post-operative care instructions. On occasions antibiotics might be prescribed.

Oral antrum fistula (OAF)

An OAF is a hole connecting the mouth and the maxillary sinus which can occur following the extraction of a tooth. This communication happens as the roots of the posterior teeth are very close to the floor of the maxillary sinus, coupled with the bone in this area being thin. In some patients the roots of the posterior teeth can actually be in the maxillary sinus. If an infection, cysts or other pathology is present it will weaken the bone around the roots of the tooth being extracted, making a communication more likely to occur.

Small openings are very common and these will normally heal by themselves without any treatment being provided. In fact, quite frequently neither the maxillofacial surgeon nor the patient is aware that the hole is present.

If an OAF is suspected the maxillofacial surgeon will ask the patient to hold their nose and blow. If an OAF is present, a bubbling of blood will occur at the extraction site. It is important that the dental nurse does not aspirate this area to avoid clot removal.

To repair an OAF the maxillofacial surgeon will raise buccal and palatal flaps. They will stretch them across the socket site and suture them with several stitches so that they will hold in place. This procedure can prove difficult, and may have to be repeated. The success of the healing process will depend upon how well the mouth is cared for in the following days. The patient will be provided with the normal post-operative care advice and be told to try to avoid blowing their nose or sneezing. If they do either of these, the suture will break open. If a non-absorbable suture is used, the patient will require another appointment 14 days later to have the sutures removed.

Loss of a tooth

On very rare occasions, an extracted tooth may be lost from vision and could be misplaced. If this occurs, it is important to establish where it is as it could possibly have fallen from the forceps to the ground or been inhaled or swallowed by the patient. The maxillofacial team would start by reassuring the patient and asking them to slowly sit up and spit into a receptor. The patient may be asked to place their head over to one side to avoid the tooth going further back into the oropharynx. If it is not in the patient's mouth, they would search the floor, ask the patient to look in their clothing and, if the practice has the facility to do so, in the suction tubing/pot by X-raying it.

If the tooth cannot be found the patient is sent for a chest/abdominal radiograph. If the tooth has passed into the alimentary canal, then no further treatment is required as it will not cause any harm. If, on the other hand, the tooth has been inhaled into the airway or lungs, an emergency operation is required to remove it before it can cause any serious complications such as pneumonia or a lung abscess. If the tooth were to be inhaled into the lungs, the one it would most likely fall into would be the right lung due to the anatomical structure route being straighter and the diaphragm being higher on this side.

Fracture of a tooth (retained roots)

During the removal of a tooth roots can be retained. This may happen for various reasons, such as the crown could de-coronate as the tooth is very carious or the roots are curved and the tip of the apex may remain in situ. When this occurs the maxillofacial surgeon will discuss the treatment options with the patient and record the conversations held in the notes. The options available are:

- To elevate the root.
- To surgically remove the root if elevation fails.
- To leave the retained root in place where it will either stagnate in the bone or eventually work its way out. This option might be considered if the root is too close to the sinus or mandibular nerve, and removing it could cause further complications. It could also be that it is firmly attached to the bone (ankyloses). The problem leaving retained roots in place is that they infect. If this action is taken, regular reviews should be carried out and X-rays taken to ensure the root is not causing any problems.

Careful appraisal of the tooth or teeth to be extracted including the taking of X-rays can help to avoid the occurrence of retained roots. The procedure is similar to that of a surgical removal of an impacted wisdom tooth. A gingival flap is raised. If the root is not visible, bone is removed. The root is then elevated or lifted out with either an elevator, Fickling's toothed forceps (Figure 5.24) or upper permanent root extraction forceps (Figure 5.5). Any bone fragments are smoothed off and the socket is irrigated with a 0.9% sodium chloride solution. The flap is then repositioned and sutured. Haemostasis is achieved and the patient provided with written and verbal post-operative care advice.

Accidental extraction

Accidental extraction can happen; however, it is fortunately rare due to protocols being formulated by maxillofacial surgeries. These can be as simple as checking the tooth to be removed with another trained professional, who quite often is the dental nurse, or having a checklist form in place. In the event that the wrong tooth is extracted, it should be replaced immediately. A splint is made to hold the tooth in position while it heals. In some cases, further treatment is needed at a later stage. Naturally the patient is advised, it is recorded in their notes and a risk assessment is carried out to prevent it happening again.

Damage to a neighbouring tooth

On occasions during the extraction of a tooth, the adjacent tooth can become damaged. It could be that a crown has been dislodged or the restoration has been chipped or fractured. Irrespective of the damage, it has to be rectified at no additional cost to the patient so that their mouth is restored to its original oral health.

Paresthesia (numbness)

Wisdom teeth sit very close to or on the nerves that supply sensation to the teeth, gingiva, cheek, lip and tongue. During their extraction these nerves can become damaged, resulting in a tingling sensation and numbness. In most cases the nerve will repair itself in a short time. In less than 2% of cases, it will be permanent. The nerves may also be numb due to swelling that has occurred as a result of the surgery. In this instance, anti-inflammatory drugs are prescribed. If lingual nerve damage occurs, patients can experience difficulty using their mouth for several weeks until it accommodates to the change. The nerve can take up to several months to repair. It is not common that this numbness will be permanent; however, it is a possibility. If the nerve was actually severed during surgery then the damage will more than likely be permanent. To prevent nerve damage the lingual nerve must be protected when the hand-piece is being used to remove bone. This is undertaken by the placement of a Howarth's periosteal elevator (Figure 5.21a). If the periosteal elevator is moved or misplaced during the procedure, the maxillofacial surgeon must be informed at once in order for it to be replaced immediately. During the consent process before extraction takes place, the patient will be warned of the possibility of nerve damage.

Weakening of the jaw

This can arise when removing impacted teeth. It is very rare, but if it does happen it will make the jaw more susceptible to fractures in the future.

Medical emergency

Patients can suffer a medical emergency at any time, irrespective of their medical history. Because maxillofacial treatments are bloodletting procedures which can last for long periods, the risk of a medical emergency is increased. All staff must be trained in dealing with the collapsed patient and be conversant with the current resuscitation procedures in force.

EXTRACTIONS

SURGICAL REMOVAL OF IMPACTED TEETH

Impacted teeth are common. They are mainly associated with the third permanent molars, which are also known as the wisdom teeth. When discussing impacted teeth, the maxillofacial surgeon will refer to the angles of impaction:

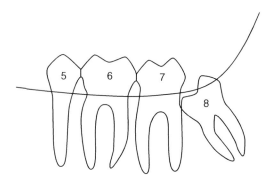

Figure 5.20 Mesio-angular impacted lower third molar. Source: Hollins, C. 2013 *Levison's Textbook for Dental Nurses*, 11th Edition, p. 545. Reproduced with permission of John Wiley & Sons.

- Vertical.
- Horizontal.
- Disto-angular.
- Mesio-angular.

The most common type of impaction is mesio-angular (Figure 5.20), as it is natural for teeth to drift towards the mesial aspect of the mouth.

The removal of an impacted wisdom tooth will necessitate a surgical procedure. This can be as simple as raising a flap and elevating the tooth. On occasions the tooth has to be segmented (split) and removed in two or more pieces.

Procedure

Prior to the removal of an impacted tooth the maxillofacial surgeon will take the appropriate X-ray to aid diagnosis and treatment planning. They will discuss the options with the patient in order for them to give consent. This will include methods of pain and anxiety control. Once consent has been taken the patient may or may not have the tooth removed that day. If the patient is asked to attend another appointment for the removal of the impacted tooth, they will be provided with pre-operative verbal and written instructions. If the patient has the impacted tooth removed on that appointment, they are provided with post-operative care instructions.

On the day of the removal of the impacted tooth consent will be checked, along with the patient's identity. The patient's medical history is re-checked and any changes noted. Personal protective equipment will be placed on the patient and a brief explanation of the procedure provided. For pain and anxiety control the clinician may apply a topical anaesthetic prior to administering the local

anaesthetic. The patient is constantly monitored and reassured. The maxillofacial surgeon will ensure that the appropriate area is numb before commencing
treatment.

They will start by making an incision with a No. 15 blade on a Bard-Parker
handle (Figure 4.6). They may choose to use a disposable No. 15 scalpel blade
and handle (Figure 4.7). Once the incision has been made, a gingival flap is
raised using a Howarth's periosteal elevator (Figure 5.21a). Some maxillofacial
surgeons may choose to use a Mitchell's osteo trimmer (Figure 5.21b). The
flap is held back with a retractor, most commonly an Austin's tissue retractor
(Figure 5.22) or Bowdler-Henry retractor (Figure 5.23). If it essential to remove
some bone, a No. 6 rosehead surgical bur (Figure 4.4) is used with a straight
surgical hand-piece (Figure 4.1) that has an irrigation tube containing 0.9%
sodium chloride solution.

Once the tooth is exposed, the maxillofacial surgeon will position the
Howarth's periosteal elevator into the socket to prevent potential nerve
damage. If the maxillofacial surgeon decides the crown of the tooth requires
dividing, a No. 4 tapered or flat fissured surgical bur (Figure 4.5) is used.
Once this has taken place and the tooth has been exposed, it will be elevated
out of the socket with an elevator. A Fickling's forcep can be used to remove
the tooth from the socket as these tightly hold the loose sections of tooth
by a clamping mechanism, preventing the individual portion of tooth being
dropped (Figure 5.24). A Cryer's (Figure 5.25) or Warwick-James elevator
(Figure 5.26) are commonly used. However, many maxillofacial surgeons will
use a Coupland's chisel as an elevator, despite its primary function to detach
the periodontal membrane from the root of the tooth.

Upon removal of the tooth the maxillofacial surgeon will inspect it to ensure
it is all accounted for. They will then irrigate the socket with 0.9% sodium
chloride solution in a 5 mL sterile disposable syringe (Figure 4.2) to ensure that
all fragments are removed; they will smooth the edges of the bone with bone
rongeurs (Figure 5.27) and a bone file (Figure 5.28) to make sure there are no
rough or sharp areas left and re-irrigate the socket.

Finally, the gingival flap is sutured back into place using Kilner needle holders (Figure 5.29), an absorbable suture (Figure 4.9), Gillie's tissue dissecting
forceps (Figure 5.30), Kilner cheek retractor (Figure 5.31) and long pointed
scissors (Figure 5.32). A Lacks retractor may be used to protect the tongue
during suturing (Figure 5.33).

Once the gingival flap has been sutured into place, a rolled-up sterile swap is
placed in the socket area. The patient will be asked to bite down on the swab for
15–20 minutes to allow haemostasis to take place. During this time, the verbal
and written post-operative care instructions are provided. Once haemostasis
has been achieved, the patient is discharged and provided with further appointments if necessary.

EXTRACTIONS

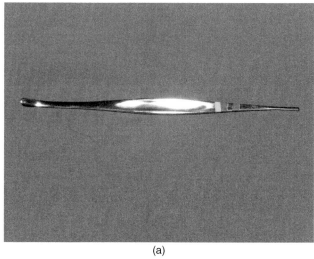

(a)

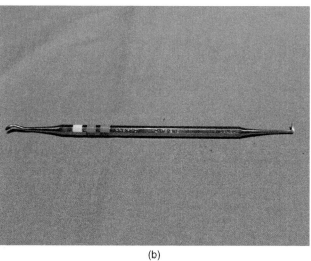

(b)

Figure 5.21 (a) Howarth's periosteal elevator. (b) Mitchell's osteo trimmer.

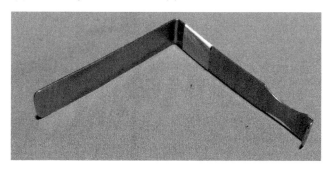

Figure 5.22 Austin's tissue retractor.

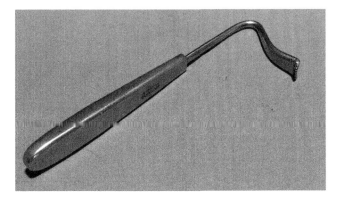

Figure 5.23 Bowdler-Henry retractor.

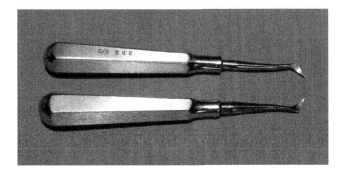

Figure 5.24 Fickling's toothed forceps.

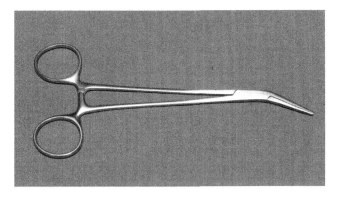

Figure 5.25 Left and right Cryer's elevator.

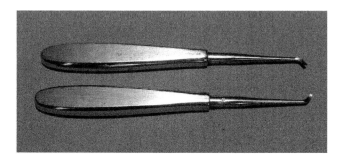

Figure 5.26 Left and right Warwick-James elevator.

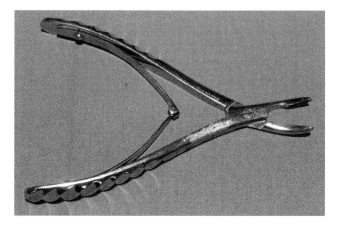

Figure 5.27 Bone rongeurs.

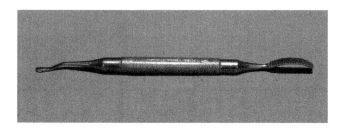

Figure 5.28 Bone file.

EXTRACTIONS

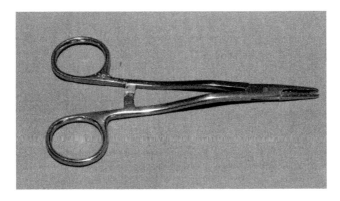

Figure 5.29 Kilner needle holders.

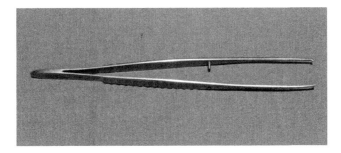

Figure 5.30 Gillie's tissue dissecting forceps.

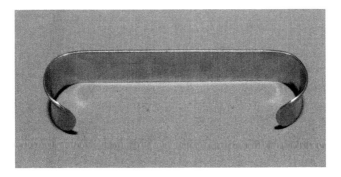

Figure 5.31 Kilner cheek retractor.

EXTRACTIONS

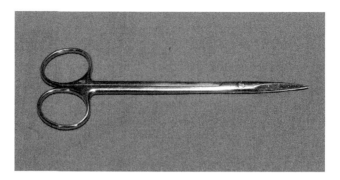

Figure 5.32 Long pointed scissors.

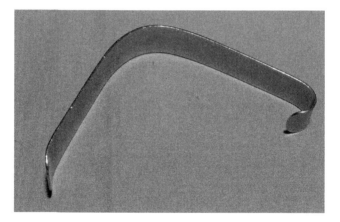

Figure 5.33 Lacks retractor.

Role of dental nurse

The dental nurse will prepare the surgery prior to the patient's arrival. They will carry out comprehensive infection control by disinfecting the primary and secondary zones and ensure that all instruments, materials and medicaments required for the planned surgical procedure are sterile. They will collect the patient's notes or ensure they are ready on the computer and display the radiographs. They will note the patient's medical history to establish if there are any special requirements for the patient and check that consent has been taken.

The dental nurse will collect the patient from the waiting room, checking that they have the correct patient and introduce themselves. They will ask them if they have eaten and adhered to the pre-operative instructions provided at the last appointment, and if they have any medication they would like placed on the work surface. They will take the patient's coat and belongings and ask them to take a seat in the dental chair.

EXTRACTIONS

Once the patient is settled they will apply the personal protective equipment in the form of a bib and glasses, explaining to the patient the rationale for each. When requested, they will scrub in readiness to prepare the items required for the maxillofacial surgeon with the help of a circulation nurse. The role of a circulation nurse is to open and drop items required onto a designated surgical field. Throughout the procedure, constant aspiration using a Yankeur suction tube (Figure 4.16) and retraction of soft tissues, as required, will take place. The passing of instruments at the correct stage of the procedure, ensuring a sterile field, will follow.

The dental nurse will hold the Howarth's periosteal elevator *in situ*. Continual reassurance and monitoring of the patient's vital signs will be undertaken. The maxillofacial surgeon may request the dental nurse to cut the sutures when being placed. They will also ensure excellent cross-infection control and the health and safety of all. If requested, the dental nurse may provide verbal and written post-operative care instructions. Once the patient has left, they will dispose of the waste correctly and carry out infection control procedures in the form of disinfection and sterilisation, returning the patient's notes and radiographs to file.

Disposal of teeth

Teeth can either be given to the patient or placed in a specialised tooth pot containing powder. If the tooth contains amalgam, the tooth would be placed in a separate pot. Both would be collected by an authorised waste contractor.

SUMMARY OF THE ROLE OF THE DENTAL NURSE

- Decontamination procedures as per HTM01-05 recommendations.
- Preparing and maintaining the clinical environment to reflect the maxillofacial procedure being undertaken.
- Ensuring the health and safety of all.
- Monitoring and reassuring the patient.
- Delivering pre- and post-operative instructions.
- Supporting the patient's head during extractions.
- Four-handed dentistry.
- Aspiration.
- Retraction of soft tissues.
- Cutting sutures.
- Process and mount radiographs.
- Taking payments.
- Book any follow-up appointments.

EXTRACTIONS

RADIOGRAPHS USED FOR EXTRACTIONS

- Dental periapical (Figure 5.34): This view is taken as it will show the whole tooth, including the apex and surrounding bone, allowing the maxillofacial surgeon to assess the apical condition of a tooth for any abscesses or other pathology present. They can also view any root fractures that may have been sustained.
- Dental panoramic tomograph (DPT) (Figure 5.35): This view is taken as it will show all the anterior and posterior teeth, both erupted and un-erupted. It will also show the temporomandibular joint, the maxillary sinus, any tumours, cysts or other pathology, retained roots, jaw fractures, missing teeth and supernumerary teeth.
- Oblique lateral: This view is taken when a patient is unable to stand still for the required time for a DPT to be taken. The right and left side of the face are taken to show all erupted and un-erupted posterior teeth, cysts, tumours, root fragments and fractures.

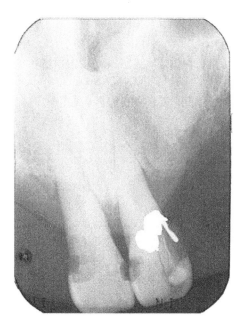

Figure 5.34 Periapical radiograph. Source: Hollins, C. 2013 *Levison's Textbook for Dental Nurses*, 11th Edition, p. 332. Reproduced with permission of John Wiley & Sons.

EXTRACTIONS

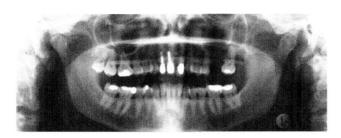

Figure 5.35 Dental panoramic tomography. Source: Hollins, C. 2013 *Levison's Textbook for Dental Nurses*, 11th Edition, p. 333. Reproduced with permission of John Wiley & Sons.

Soft tissue lesions and conditions of the mouth, and methods of their investigation

At the end of this chapter you should have an understanding of:

1. Soft tissue lesions and conditions of the mouth.
2. Biopsies.

LESIONS AND CONDITIONS OF THE MOUTH

Fibroepithelial polyp (FEP)

These are common, benign, slow-growing fibrous lumps (Figure 6.1) which are usually painless. Fibroepithelial polyps are usually caused by trauma or from a source of irritation to the soft tissues such as a sharp tooth or cheek biting. They are often seen in adults, commonly presenting on the tongue, buccal mucosa and lips. They have the appearance of a shiny, smooth, round lump. Fibroepithelial polyps may attach to the mucosa by either a stalk or at the base of the lump itself. Fibroepithelial polyps may also present on the palate as a flattened lesion known as leaf fribroma. These palatal lesions usually occur under an ill-fitting denture.

Basic Guide to Oral and Maxillofacial Surgery, First Edition. Nicola Rogers and Cinzia Pickett.
© 2017 John Wiley & Sons Ltd. Published 2017 by John Wiley & Sons Ltd.

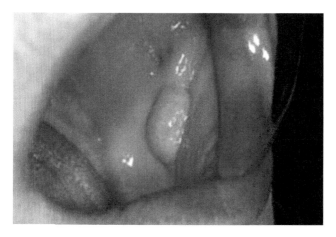

Figure 6.1 Fibrous lump. Source: Pedro Diz Dios, Crispian Scully, Oslei Paes de Almeida, Jose V. Bagán, Adalberto Mosqueda Taylor, 2016. *Oral Medicine and Pathology at a Glance*, 2nd Edition, p. 48. Reproduced with permission of John Wiley & Sons.

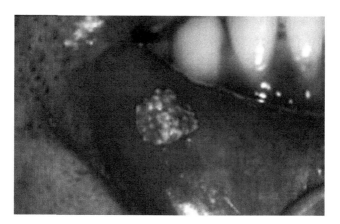

Figure 6.2 Papilloma. Source: Pedro Diz Dios, Crispian Scully, Oslei Paes de Almeida, Jose V. Bagán, Adalberto Mosqueda Taylor, 2016. *Oral Medicine and Pathology at a Glance*, 2nd Edition, p. 44. Reproduced with permission of John Wiley & Sons.

Papilloma

These present as small, benign, cauliflower-like lesions which are usually white or pink in colour. Papillomas (Figure 6.2) are most commonly found on the tongue, lips, buccal mucosa or on the palate, particularly where the hard and soft palate join. Papillomas are caused by a type of human papilloma virus (HPV); however, this type of papilloma appears to be benign as opposed to other types of papillomas in the body which may become malignant.

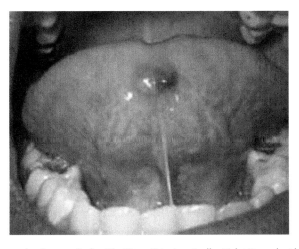

Figure 6.3 Mucocele. Source: Pedro Diz Dios, Crispian Scully, Oslei Paes de Almeida, Jose V. Bagán, Adalberto Mosqueda Taylor, 2016. *Oral Medicine and Pathology at a Glance*, 2nd Edition, p. 82. Reproduced with permission of John Wiley & Sons.

Mucocele (mucus cyst/mucus extravasation cyst)

Mucoceles (Figure 6.3) are painless, translucent, smooth, soft swellings. They may vary in size, and can be up to 1–2 cm in diameter. They commonly occur on the inside of the lower lip, but may also occur on the ventrum of the tongue, floor of mouth and occasionally the palate. Mucoceles may appear slightly bluish/white in colour. These lesions are usually attributed to trauma of a minor salivary gland, for example accidentally biting the lip. When recording the history of the lesion during the assessment appointment, the patient may explain that the swelling ruptures from time to time then recurs. Many patients wish to have these lesions removed as the position of the mucocele, particularly on the lower lip, may be troublesome to the patient particularly when eating; further trauma may also occur through accidental biting of the lesion. However, if the mucocele is small and not troublesome they may be left and kept under observation. If they are removed, as with all soft tissue lesions the sample should be sent to pathology for a histology report to confirm diagnosis.

Haemangioma

Haemangiomas are vascular lesions consisting of malformed blood vessels. These lesions appear as flat red, purple or bluish areas usually occurring on the lip, buccal mucosa, palate or tongue. As haemangiomas are vascular they are soft and compressible, and blanch upon pressure. They are frequently left due to the complication of haemorrhage associated with their removal.

SOFT TISSUE LESIONS AND
CONDITIONS OF THE MOUTH

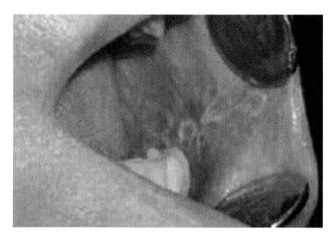

Figure 6.4 Lichen planus. Source: Pedro Diz Dios, Crispian Scully, Oslei Paes de Almeida, Jose V. Bagán, Adalberto Mosqueda Taylor, 2016. *Oral Medicine and Pathology at a Glance,* 2nd Edition, p. 70. Reproduced with permission of John Wiley & Sons.

Lichen planus

Lichen planus (Figure 6.4) is usually symptomless; however, some patients suffer from painful flare-ups which can be troublesome, affecting the patient's ability to eat and drink, and can be distressing at times. It is a common condition that, orally, can affect areas of the buccal mucosa, tongue, floor of mouth and gingiva. It is distinguishable by its white lace-like patterns and/or red, angry, erosive areas. Confirmation of suspected lichen planus is usually carried out by performing a biopsy. Although there is no 'cure' for any confirmed diagnosis, it is important that more serious conditions are ruled out through histopathology investigation. Lichen planus is a persistent condition and although there is no definitive treatment, the condition is usually symptom free. During any flare-ups, a steroid mouthwash may shorten the duration of any painful, troublesome episodes. Patients who suffer with lichen planus are kept under review and, if the presentation of the lesion changes, a further biopsy may be performed.

Geographic tongue

Geographic tongue is a common, benign, inflammatory condition. It commonly affects the dorsum area of the tongue. It may be asymptomatic but for some patients it can cause soreness, particularly when eating acidic or spicy food as this can make the condition worse. Geographic tongue is a non-contagious condition. Areas of depapillation develop, leaving areas of erythema (red). These smooth, red patches are irregular in shape, size and may give the appearance of a map-like pattern on the tongue. These areas can spread, move or change within days or weeks and may even spontaneously resolve only for a new area to appear in a new location on the tongue. The cause of geographic tongue is unknown, but there has been suggestion that it may be linked to a genetic predisposition as it is a condition that tends to run in families. There is no specific treatment. Many people with geographic tongue find that avoiding certain foods helps to control the condition. For any soreness or discomfort, over–the-counter analgesics or a non-steroidal anti-inflammatory may be used. An anaesthetic mouthwash may prove helpful and, on occasions, corticosteroids and zinc supplements.

Oral candidiasis

Also known as oral thrush, oral candidiasis is a fungal infection of the mouth. It may appear as a white patch which can be removed by gentle rubbing to reveal an area of redness. Its development may be associated with factors including poor oral hygiene, medications such as steroidal inhalers, antibiotic therapy and also diabetes and xerostomia. Patients may be unaware of its presence within the mouth as it can be symptomless. Some however may experience discomfort, a burning sensation or an unpleasant taste (dysgeusia). Treatment may include the use of anti-fungal medication and mitigation of the primary factors causing the condition.

Ulcers

These are common, self-limiting, shallow, circular lesions with a white/yellow area surrounded by a red border which may be slightly raised. Ulcers may present individually or as a cluster of several lesions. Individual ulcers are usually caused by trauma to the oral tissues. Many are painful and tender which may cause transient difficulties with oral hygiene, eating, drinking, speaking and swallowing. As there is no curative treatment for ulcers, management of the condition involves ameliorating any pain or discomfort while allowing the lesion to heal.

Ulcers (also known as aphthae, aphthous or aphthosis) may be attributed to trauma, anxiety, stress, systemic disease and possible deficiencies in some vitamins. Ulcers may also be linked to hormonal changes and a genetic predisposition. Recurrent episodes of ulceration may indicate a need for further investigation, and haematological analysis by routine blood screening can exclude any underlying deficiencies, particularly in iron, folic and B12 levels.

Minor aphthae
- Less than 10 mm in diameter.
- Self-limiting/-healing within 7–10 days.
- Heals without scarring.

Major aphthae
- A diameter greater than 10 mm.
- Longer lasting.
- Painful, deep lesions that when healed leave scarring.

Referral
Although ulcers are usually self-limiting, should an underlying cause of the ulceration be suspected referral to a specialist for further investigation may be necessary. Any unexplained ulceration of the oral mucosa, tongue or gingiva persisting for more than 3 weeks should be urgently referred to the maxillofacial consultant.

Burning mouth syndrome

Burning mouth syndrome is also sometimes referred to as glossodynia. Burning mouth syndrome (BMS) is characterised by a burning pain in the mouth which has no obvious cause. The pain can be localised, affecting areas of the tongue, lip, palate or gingiva or widespread, involving large areas of the mouth. There are many known factors which may be attributed to BMS, but it can be difficult to determine the definitive cause. These underlying factors may include:

- Low levels of iron, folic acid and vitamin B12.
- Oral candidiasis.
- Xerostomia.
- Gastric reflux.
- Neuropathy.
- Hormonal changes.
- Allergic reaction.
- Stress, anxiety and depression.

Blood tests and a microbiology swab may disclose an underlying cause which, when treated, will resolve the symptoms of BMS. However, BMS may unfortunately be a long-term condition. Medication may be offered to help patients cope with the chronic pain.

Trigeminal neuralgia

As described in Chapter 2 the Vth cranial nerve, the trigeminal nerve, has three divisions: ophthalmic, maxillary and mandibular branches. Trigeminal neuralgia is a dysfunction of this nerve. It may be idiopathic or related to demyelination disease such as multiple sclerosis. Dysfunction of the trigeminal nerve causes the individual to have severe facial pain. The extreme pain may be intermittent and described as an intense burning, electric shock or stabbing pain. Trigeminal neuralgia is a long-term condition with periods of remission. Treatment involves controlling symptoms and may include analgesics, anti-convulsants and anti-depressant medications.

Bell's palsy

Usually effecting one side of the face, Bell's palsy is the most common cause of sudden facial paralysis. It is characterised by weakness of the facial muscles caused by a dysfunction of the facial nerve (VIIth cranial nerve). It is thought that inflammation of this nerve and its subsequent swelling cause a compression of the nerve which in turn causes the facial weakness. Steroid treatment to reduce the inflammation and swelling usually results in complete recovery; however, some patients may unfortunately have long-term problems.

Leukoplakia

Leukoplakia ('white plaque') is the clinical term for a white patch which does not fit any other diagnosis of lesion or disease. Usually painless, these persistent patches cannot be wiped off and, although they may be harmless, further investigation by biopsy with a histopathology report is warranted. This is attributed to the increased risk that these areas may contain abnormal cells (dysplasia). Laser ablation may be used to remove areas of dysplasia when there is a high risk that the lesion could turn malignant. The histopathology report may show hyperkeratosis, a thickening of the mucosal membrane. This is usually caused in reaction to an irritant such as smoking, alcohol consumption or friction. In these cases, further advice regarding mitigation of the source of the irritation may be necessary.

Erythroplakia

A red patch ('red plaque') which may bleed easily is less commonly seen than leukoplakia; unfortunately, however, it is more likely to become cancerous. It is estimated that around 50% of erythroplakia lesions become malignant. As with leukoplakia, a biopsy may be necessary with further treatment and regular follow-up appointments.

Orofacial cancer

Cancer is the uncontrolled growth of abnormal cells. Cancers which may be diagnosed and treated can include skin, sinus, lymphoma, salivary gland and oral. It is important to remember that some tumours are non-cancerous and do not spread; these are classified as benign (described further in Chapter 7).

SOFT TISSUE LESIONS AND
CONDITIONS OF THE MOUTH

Xerostomia

A dry mouth can occur through dehydration and nervousness; this is however normally short lived and easily resolved. Xerostomia is a condition caused by absent or reduced saliva flow or a change in the saliva's composition. Xerostomia may be idiopathic (of unknown cause), but there are known factors which may result in an individual developing a dry mouth.

A dry mouth can be a side-effect of prescribed medications. It is a condition frequently seen in older patients where medications and a natural reduction in saliva production may lead to xerostomia. Medications such as tricyclic anti-depressants, beta-blocker and anti-epileptic drugs list a dry mouth as a possible common side-effect.

Radiotherapy treatment to the head or neck and Sjögren's syndrome may also cause xerostomia.

METHODS OF INVESTIGATION

Biopsy

A biopsy is the surgical removal of tissue so that it may be microscopically investigated. It involves removing a small piece of tissue that is sent to a pathology laboratory for a pathologist to examine it under a microscope (histology). A soft-tissue biopsy is often used in maxillofacial and oral surgery and is the most common type used in the detection of oral cancer. Biopsies are a straightforward procedure and do not take very long to perform. Samples of tissue can be taken from the lips, cheeks, tongue, gingivae and skin. A biopsy can be incisional or excisional.

- **Incisional biopsy**: An incisional biopsy is where the maxillofacial surgeon will make an incision through half of the affected tissue and take an equal part of unaffected tissue. This will allow the two areas to be compared.
- **Excisional biopsy**: An excisional biopsy (Figure 6.5) is where the maxillofacial surgeon makes an incision around all of the affected area.

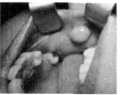 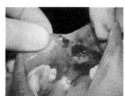 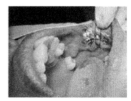

Figure 6.5 Excision of lump. Source: Pedro Diz Dios, Crispian Scully, Oslei Paes de Almeida, Jose V. Bagán, Adalberto Mosqueda Taylor, 2016. *Oral Medicine and Pathology at a Glance*, 2nd Edition, p. 6. Reproduced with permission of John Wiley & Sons.

SOFT TISSUE LESIONS AND CONDITIONS OF THE MOUTH

The maxillofacial surgeon will decide which type of biopsy is to be performed based on various factors. For example, if the lesion is small and not thought to be cancerous, an excisional biopsy will be carried out; however, if the lesion is large or possibly malignant/cancerous an incisional biopsy will be performed.

Procedure

Prior to a biopsy being carried out, the maxillofacial surgeon will discuss the type of biopsy to be performed with the patient and take consent, allowing the patient to ask questions. A local anaesthetic would be administered. Once the patient is numb, a No. 15 Bard-Parker scalpel blade and handle or a disposable one is used to remove the lesion. A diathermy machine or biopsy punch (Figure 6.6) can also be used. The sample of tissue will be held with Gillie's tissue-dissecting forceps. With either type of biopsy, the maxillofacial surgeon may place a suture through the sample of tissue being removed prior to performing the biopsy to secure it in place, so that it is not accidently aspirated away. This also acts as a marker, allowing the pathologist and consultant to orientate the sample once the results are known.

Upon removal, the sample of tissue is placed into a sterile pot which contains 10% formal saline (Figure 6.6). The area where the biopsy has been performed will either be sutured, left open or cauterised with silver nitrate, depending upon whether the surgery is minor or not and its location. If sutured, Kilner needle holders, an absorbable suture, Gillie's tissue-dissecting forceps, Kilner cheek retractor and long-nosed scissors are required. The patient is given an appointment to return for suture removal, although intra-oral sutures (Figure 6.6) are usually dissolvable.

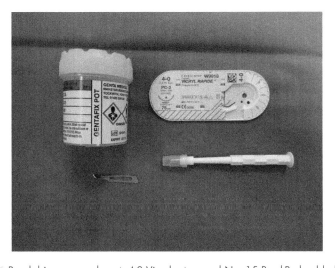

Figure 6.6 Punch biopsy, sample pot, 4-0 Vicryl suture and No. 15 Bard-Parker blade.

SOFT TISSUE LESIONS AND
CONDITIONS OF THE MOUTH

An appointment for the results of the biopsy and future treatment discussions if required is also arranged. Should an immunofluorescent examination of the tissue sample be required to assess for antibody deposits, then a specific type of histology pot and medium would be requested by the clinician; the formaldehyde in standard biopsy sample pots would render the specimen useless for this specific type of pathology reporting.

Role of dental nurse

The dental nurse's role and post-operative instructions would be the same as for any other surgical procedure, with the exception that retractors may not be used and held by the dental nurse as she/he may be requested to hold the area where the biopsy is being performed (e.g. the tongue). To prevent the oral structure slipping, holding it with sterilised gauze can help to prevent this. The gauze will also help with moisture control and, on occasions, the maxillofacial surgeon will prefer the biopsy site to be kept clear with gauze as opposed to aspiration.

Fine needle aspiration (FNA)

Fine needle aspiration (FNA) is often used for screening as the initial diagnosis for lesions of the head and neck. It is fairly accurate, quick to perform, inexpensive to undertake and patients tolerate this procedure well. Sites in the head and neck amenable to FNA include the thyroid, cervical masses and nodules, salivary glands, intraoral lesions and lesions in the paraspinal area and base of the skull. Diagnostic accuracy is dependent upon the site of aspiration, as well as the skill of the individual performing and interpreting the FNA.

Most FNA procedures are undertaken as an outpatient procedure within a maxillofacial unit. Sometimes ultrasound imagery is needed to guide the needle into the correct area and, in these cases, the aspiration will be performed within a radiography department, usually by a radiologist. This ultrasound-guided aspiration is particularly useful for head and neck masses when the mass is not palpable. They involve a thin needle being inserted into the abnormal tissue or fluid collection to take cell samples by capillary action (cells migrate/are aspirated up into the needle). It is considered to be a safe procedure as the risk of complications is fairly low. The procedure takes approximately 15 minutes.

Prior to FNA being carried out, the maxillofacial surgeon will discuss the reason for performing this biopsy with the patient and take consent, allowing the patient to ask questions.

FNA is a surgical technique and therefore aseptic techniques will be employed. Patients undergoing an FNA will have the skin surrounding the area where the procedure will be carried out wiped with a disinfectant and draped with sterile towels or disposable sheets. A local anaesthetic may be administered into the procedural area. The needle is very thin and is

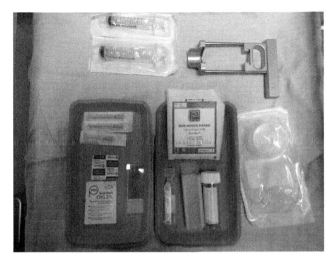

Figure 6.7 FNA instruments.

attached to a syringe that is inserted into the skin to reach the underlying area. The syringe has a vacuum that permits the bodily cells to be aspirated up into the needle and syringe (Figure 6.7). The clinician may move and reposition the needle to ensure that an adequate sample of cells is aspirated into the syringe. Once the needle is removed, pressure is applied to the area to stop any bleeding.

The sample collected can be immediately examined under a microscope to verify that the sample taken is adequate, which also provides a quick diagnosis. Some biopsy samples are dispatched to the laboratory for further analysis before the diagnostic result is provided, in which case the patient is given an appointment to return.

Microscope glass slides (Figure 6.7) are used to transport the sample to the laboratory for examination. These slides are usually 25×76 mm and approximately 1 mm in thickness. They comprise a white frosted area at one end for recording the patients name, date of birth and hospital number. The rest of the glass slide is clear glass, and it is on this clear area that the sample is applied. The aspirated sample should be carefully spread in small amounts over several glass slides to create a thin layer on each slide prior to fixation.

There are two methods commonly used: air dried and alcohol fixation. When using the air-dried method, the sample on the slide must be thin enough to ensure that the sample is to the eye dry within 5 minutes. This prevents artefacts being present during the microscopic examination. Also known as 'wet slides', any slides requiring alcohol fixation must be dipped or sprayed with ethyl immediately after the sample has been placed onto the glass slide. As pathologists may wish to use different laboratory stains on the samples during the cytology examination of the sampled cells. Many clinicians choose to fix some slides with alcohol while allowing others to air dry, therefore maximising the choice of stains available to the pathologist. The slides should then be carefully placed into plastic microscope slide boxes for safe transportation to the laboratory with the appropriately completed and labelled cytology request form. As with other pathology request forms, the information should include:

- Patient's details (name, address, date of birth, hospital number).
- The date and time of the sample collection and the requesting clinician's name and signature.
- Consultant's name or code.
- Hospital department or ward.
- Clinical information/details.

Patients may feel a little discomfort in the area where the FNA was performed and may be advised to take whatever they normally take for a headache. Other post-operative symptoms which patients may experience include slight swelling and soreness, bruising and infection, although this is rare due to the sterile techniques used.

Role of dental nurse

The dental nurse's role during fine needle aspiration depends upon the clinician's preferences. However, these may include:

- Greeting the patient.
- Monitoring and reassuring the patient.
- Ensuring that all the FNA necessary resources and equipment (Figure 6.7) are available to the clinician.
- Passing items as required.
- Accurate labelling of the glass slides.
- Providing pressure to the puncture site.
- Decontamination and cross-infection control.

Microbiology swabs

Microbiology is the study of microscopic organisms. Microbiology tests are accurate in identifying conditions affecting the oral cavity and skin. Generally, microbiology tests are performed using a microbiology swab (Figure 6.8), consisting of a swab on the end of a plastic shaft with an appropriate transport medium within a plastic tube. The swab is applied to the area under investigation and then returned to the plastic tube. The plastic tube is labelled with the patient's details. A laboratory request form is completed, containing details of the specimen, the reason for the test, the patient's details, date and time the specimen was taken, and the consultant's name and department details.

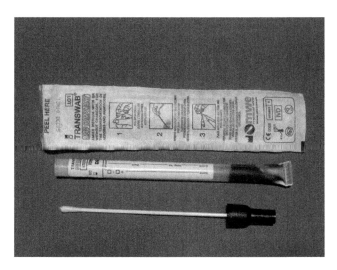

Figure 6.8 Microbiology swab.

Ultrasound

An ultrasound scan, sometimes known as a sonogram, produces an image of part of the inside of the body by using high-frequency sound waves that cannot be heard. As the waves bounce off different parts of the body echoes are produced and picked up by the probe, resulting in a moving image. The principle of an ultrasound scan is similar to sonar used by submarines.

The benefits of an ultrasound scan are that the technique can be used for all age groups and for those with medical ailments or physical disabilities. There is no radiation involvement or intravenous contrast medium used. Biopsies and drainage can be undertaken in conjunction with ultrasound scans and the resolution is better than a magnetic resonance imaging (MRI) or computerised tomography (CT) scan. They are considered to be safe; to date, there are no known risks. They are performed by a radiologist or sonographer. When a patient has an ultrasound scan they will be given specific instructions which will result in a better quality image, such as not eating. Scans can take 15–45 minutes and, in some cases, sedatives can be provided if the patient is anxious.

Ultrasound scans can be internal and external; the type used in maxillofacial surgery is external. The ultrasound scanner comprises a console, computer, viewing screen and hand-held probe coated with a lubricant. It is placed on and moved over the skin. The lubricant enables the probe to move smoothly over the skin; the only sensation the patient should experience is the sensor being moved which can sometimes feel cold. The scan appears immediately on the screen.

Following the ultrasound the patient can resume normal daily activities. If a sedative has however been provided, specific aftercare instructions must be

SOFT TISSUE LESIONS AND CONDITIONS OF THE MOUTH

adhered to (described in Chapter 3). The results of the ultrasound scan can be viewed immediately; however, most need to be viewed and reported on by a consultant radiologist. In the latter case the patient has an appointment to return.

Computerised tomograhy (CT)

X-rays and a computer are used to produce a computerised tomography (CT) scan, sometimes also known as computer-assisted tomography (CAT) scans. They produce detailed images of the inside of the body, including blood vessels, internal organs and the bones. They are performed by radiographers with extended duties and take approximately 10–20 minutes. Quite often they are undertaken when a person is an inpatient during a hospital stay, but outpatient CT scans are also undertaken.

CT scans are considered to be generally safe even though X-rays are used, as the scanners are designed to ensure that the dose of radiation received is not unnecessarily high. Naturally the amount of radiation will vary depending upon how much of the body is being scanned. It is thought that the dose of radiation received during a CT scan is comparable to several years' natural background radiation. As with dental X-rays, the benefit of having a CT scan would have to outweigh the risks involved. This would naturally be discussed with the patient.

Prior to a CT scan the patient will be given instructions to follow so that the resulting image is optimal. They will be told to wear comfortable clothes that are not tight or contain any metal fasteners or zips, and to leave jewellery at home. The patient should avoid eating for the few hours before the scan so that a clear image is obtained. Female patients will additionally be advised to inform the radiographer if they are pregnant, as a scan would only be undertaken for immediate emergency treatment.

Production of a CT scan

Prior to the CT scan the patient may be given a contrast medium (dye), either placed through an indwelling venflon which will allow the dye to enter directly into the bloodstream or in the form of a drink. There is a risk that the patient could be allergic to this dye. The radiographer will support the patient throughout the procedure and can arrange for a sedative to be administered should the patient be anxious. The patient may be requested to remove any clothing that could impede the scan and any items that contain metal as this will interfere with the scanning equipment.

The patient is laid flat on their back on a bed that moves into the scanner, which comprises rings that rotate around small sectional areas of the body as the patient passes through it. Patents should not feel claustrophobic as the scanner does not surround the whole body. The radiographer will speak through

SOFT TISSUE LESIONS AND CONDITIONS OF THE MOUTH

an intercom to the patient as they operate the scanner in another room. They will ask the patient to breathe normally, lie still and may at certain points ask them to breathe in and out or even to hold their breath.

Once the scan has been taken the patient can return home and resume normal daily activities, provided that a dye has not been administered. If a dye was used, then the patient would be kept for an hour or so to ensure that no reaction takes place. Upon discharge, the patient would be informed that the dye will pass through while urinating. The results of a scan will be viewed, interpreted and reported by a radiologist and are usually ready to discuss with the referring clinician within a few weeks.

Magnetic resonance imaging (MRI)

A magnetic resonance imaging (MRI) scan is a medical investigation that uses exceptionally strong magnetic and radio-frequency waves to generate images of the body. To take and produce an MRI scan, a patient lies flat in a large tube which contains very powerful magnets. The scan uses strong magnetic fields and radio waves to create detailed images of the inside of the body, the results of which can help to diagnose the patient's condition. They can be used to scan nearly every part of the body.

MRI scans are safe as they do not involve any radiation. One of the problems with an MRI scan is that the patient has to lie still in a small tube. This may prove difficult for some patients, such as those who suffer from claustrophobia. MRI scans are taken by radiographers with extended duties who support the patient through the process. Ear plugs are given to patients through which music is piped to block out the tapping noise that the scanner will periodically make. They also provide a means for the radiographer to communicate with the patient.

The patient may be placed in the MRI scanner either feet or head first, depending upon the area of the body under investigation. Once the patient has been moved into the MRI scanner, the radiographer will control the scanner via a computer situated in a different room. The reason for the computer being in another room is so that it will not be affected by the magnetic field that the scanner will generate while scanning the patient. The radiographer can watch the patient on a television monitor to ensure they are lying still, comfortable and not moving or experiencing any difficulties. Depending upon the amount of images required and the size of the area being scanned, an MRI scan can take approximately 15–90 minutes.

Not all patients can have an MRI, for example patients with pacemakers fitted or those with any metal plates in their bodies would be contraindicated. Pregnant patients or those breast-feeding should advise the radiographer prior to an MRI scan; although there is to date no evidence stating that MRI scans are harmful, they are not recommended during the first trimester.

SOFT TISSUE LESIONS AND
CONDITIONS OF THE MOUTH

Production of an MRI scan

The human body mainly comprises water molecules that contain hydrogen and oxygen atoms. The centre of the hydrogen atom contains small particles called protons. Since protons are comparable to tiny magnets, they are sensitive to magnetic fields. When a patient is in the MRI scanner, these photons will line up with the powerful magnets inside the tube. The protons are knocked out of alignment by short blasts of radio waves being sent to specific areas of the body. When the radio waves cease, the protons realign with the powerful magnets. This results in radio signals being transmitted and received. It is through these signals that information is obtained about the precise location of the protons, including distinction between different types of tissues within the body. The signals received from the protons combine to provide a detailed image of the inside of the body. MRI scanning produces an image in the form of a slice of the patient's body, where the slice can be as thin as a couple of millimetres and can be in any direction. These images are viewed, interpreted and reported upon by a radiologist.

Chapter 7

Trauma and complex procedures

At the end of this chapter you should have a clear understanding of:

1. Trauma.
2. Temporomandibular joint disorder.
3. Salivary gland surgery.
4. Craniofacial and oral cancer.
5. Cleft lip and palate.
6. Bisphosphonate-related osteonecrosis of the jaw (BRONJ).
7. Anticoagulant therapy.
8. Orthognathic surgery.
9. Dental implants.
10. Tongue-tie release.
11. Apicectomy.
12. Avulsion.
13. Alveolectomy.
14. The role of the dental nurse during complex procedures.

TRAUMA

Frequently, the maxillofacial outpatient team will be requested to assess and treat patients who have suffered trauma to the face, head or neck. There is a wide spectrum of severity of injuries that may be encountered ranging from cuts, bruising and bites to complex lacerations, fractures and high-velocity injuries. Factors and situations that may be associated with traumatic injuries are alcohol consumption and associated behaviour, sports injuries, falls and disease.

Basic Guide to Oral and Maxillofacial Surgery, First Edition. Nicola Rogers and Cinzia Pickett.
© 2017 John Wiley & Sons Ltd. Published 2017 by John Wiley & Sons Ltd.

Patients who have suffered traumatic injuries will usually be referred to the maxillofacial department by either accident and emergency (A&E), medical assessment unit (MAU) or a hospital ward. Prior to this referral, initial assessment and stabilisation of the patient's overall condition will have been carried out. This may include:

- Airway, breathing and circulation assessment (ABC).
- Initial assessment of injuries, including possible head injury.
- Assessment and treatment of other injuries.
- Imagery (radiographs, CT and MRI scans).
- Pain control.
- Prophylaxis antibiotics.

Once the referral has been received by the maxillofacial department, the patient will be assessed by a team member who will then either treat the patient if the injury is within their scope of practice or, if needed, refer to a consultant maxillofacial surgeon.

Fractures

Trauma such as a fall, assault, sporting or road traffic accident (RTA) may cause injury to the facial bones. Fractures caused by a trauma are classified as simple, compound or comminuted:

- **Simple:** There are several types of simple fractures; however, in all cases the fractured bone does not penetrate the skin.
- **Compound:** The fractured bone penetrates the surrounding tissues and skin and is exposed to the external environment.
- **Comminuted:** With a comminuted fracture the bone fractures into several fragments.

Fractures of the mandible

Fractures of the mandible, caused by trauma to the lower face, are frequently seen within the maxillofacial department. Mandibular fractures may be unilateral (affecting one side), bilateral (affecting both sides) or multiple. These fractures are classified (Figure 7.1) as being:

- **Condylar:** a fracture of the condyle, either unilateral or bilateral.
- **Coronoid:** a fracture of the coronoid process which will usually involve fractures to other neighbouring structures.
- **Angle:** a fracture where separation of the ramus and body occurs.
- **Ramus:** a fracture between the angle of the mandible and the condylar area.
- **Body:** a fracture between the angle and the parasymphyseal.
- **Symphyseal:** a mid-line fracture.

TRAUMA AND COMPLEX PROCEDURES

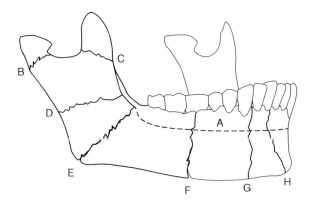

Figure 7.1 Classification of mandibular fracture sites. A, dentoalveolar; B, condylar; C, coronoid; D, ramus; E, angle; F, body (molar/premolar area); G, parasymphysis; H, symphysis.

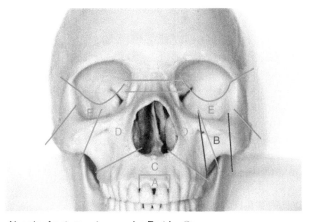

Alveolar fracture – A;	Le Fort I – C;
Molar fracture of	Le Fort II – D;
cheek bone – B;	Le Fort III – E.

Figure 7.2 Maxillary fractures. A, alveolar; B, molar fracture of cheek bone; C, Le Fort I; D, Le Fort II; E, Le Fort III. Source: Hollins, C. 2012. *Basic Guide to Anatomy and Physiology for Dental Care Professionals*, p.116. Reproduced with permission of John Wiley & Sons.

- **Parasymphyseal:** a vertical fracture in the region of the lower canine area.
- **Dentoalveolar:** a fracture of the alveolar bone.

Fractures of the mid-face
Fractures involving the mid-face region (Figure 7.2) are categorised as.

- **Le Fort I:** A horizontal fracture above the maxillary teeth. This fracture in effect separates the upper jaw from the face and is sometimes referred to as a 'floating palate'.

- **Le Fort II:** A pyramid-shaped fracture involving the orbital rims and nose.
- **Le Fort III:** A high-level horizontal fracture which traverses through several structures including the orbits, ethmoid and zygomatic arches. This complex fracture separates the whole of the mid-face from the cranium.

Injury to the mid-face may result in a fracture to the zygomatic process. This injury is usually attributed to a form of blunt trauma such as an assault. Fractures to this area involve the orbit. Fractures to the orbital floor are sometimes referred to as an 'orbital blow-out'. As with any fracture there are different levels of severity. Simple fractures which are non-displaced may heal uneventfully. More complex fractures which are displaced, or if tissue from surrounding structures is entrapped, may require surgical intervention.

Patients presenting with this injury may complain of double vision (diplopia). There may also be a flattening of the face in the cheekbone area; however, due to swelling following injury this may not be initially noticeable.

Treatment

All bone fractures need time to heal and this usually involves some form of immobilisation. For fractures of the face this can be challenging. Some fractures which are un-displaced may be suitable for conservative treatment. This would involve a prescribed period of eating soft food, rest, analgesics, good oral hygiene and refraining from contact sports. Some unilateral condylar fractures may be suitable for this form of treatment.

Should the fracture be displaced or complex, the maxillofacial surgeon will aim to realign, restore and maintain alignment of the fracture. This is referred to as reduction and fixation.

Inter-maxillary fixation (IMF)

This is a form of indirect fixation and may be suitable for some simple fractures. IMF uses arch bars and wires to secure the upper and lower jaws together. IMF aims to maintain the patient's occlusion, thus immobilising the fracture indirectly. Although IMF treatment alone does avoid the need for an open surgical procedure, it is not without its own disadvantages. IMF prolongs the patient's convalescence, and the patient will only be able to eat a liquid or semi-liquid diet for a number of weeks. It is also likely that, due to the nature of IMF, the individual's oral hygiene will deteriorate during treatment as they will not be able to clean sufficiently well.

Open reduction and internal fixation (ORIF)

When reduction and stabilisation of the fracture is needed, direct fixation may be necessary. Intervention known as ORIF (Figure 7.3) will be performed. This is a surgical procedure performed by the surgeon in theatre with the patient under general anaesthesia. Exposure to the fracture site is usually gained intra-orally; however, there may be a requirement for an external

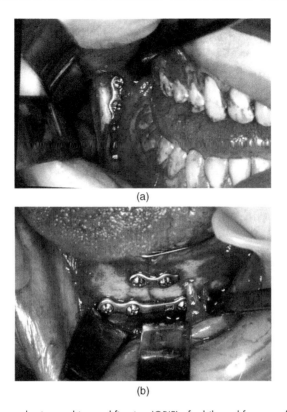

(a)

(b)

Figure 7.3 Open reduction and internal fixation (ORIF) of a bilateral fracture of the mandible using an intraoral approach and titanium miniplates with monocortical screws. Source: Michael Perry, Andrew Brown, Peter Banks, 2015. *Fractures of the Facial Skeleton*, 2nd Edition, p. 74. Reproduced with permission of John Wiley & Sons.

incision. The fracture will be reduced and fixed into a stable position with plates, screws and wires. The patient may in some cases require IMF. Upon discharge analgesics will be prescribed and the patient will be advised of the recommended post-operative instructions, which may be similar to those given for conservative treatment.

Soft tissue

Soft tissue injuries which may be treated within the maxillofacial department may include lacerations, bites, bruising and haematomas involving the head, face or neck. Following initial assessment and stabilisation, patients may be referred to the maxillofacial surgeon for definitive treatment. It is important to remember that the patient may require much reassurance as they may be quite understandably concerned and distressed.

Lacerations and bites

Lacerations and bites can vary in size and severity. Some may appear initially superficial, but careful examination may disclose complications such as a deep shelf laceration and 'through-and-through' wounds which may involve underlying blood vessels, nerves and muscles. Lacerations and bites to the face may involve anatomical boundaries such as around the lip and eye which will require precise realignment during its repair. Through-and-through lacerations (Figure 7.4) penetrate skin and tissue through to the mucosa of the mouth.

Before definitive closure of the injury is performed, thorough cleaning and debridement of the area to remove possible debris is essential. Sterile solution

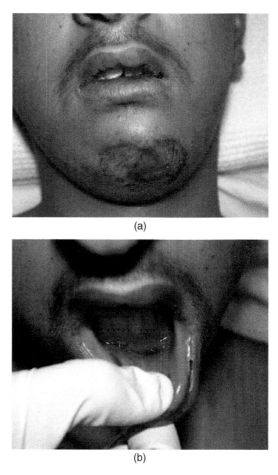

(a)

(b)

Figure 7.4 (a) 'Through-and-through' laceration of the chin. (b) What may appear on cursory examination to be a superficial injury actually extends through all layers to the oral cavity. Careful cleaning prior to repair is essential. Source: Michael Perry, Andrew Brown, Peter Banks, 2015. *Fractures of the Facial Skeleton*, 2nd Edition, p. 128. Reproduced with permission of John Wiley & Sons.

is used to irrigate the wound and any visible debris and foreign objects must be carefully removed by the clinician; this will prevent tattooing once healing has occurred. Gentle scrubbing using a soft bristled brush such as a toothbrush may also be used.

Once the area has been thoroughly cleaned, absorbable sutures are placed in the deeper tissue first. These sutures bring the involved deeper tissues together, aiding healing. Following this, monofilament, non-absorbable sterile sutures are placed in the skin to completely close the wound. The clinician may place a dressing over the area; this is not always necessary, however. An antibacterial ointment may also be prescribed for the patient to apply as directed. As the sutures are non-absorbable, the patient will need to attend a follow-up appointment for these to be removed. This will also provide a good opportunity for healing to be monitored.

Bruises
Bruising is caused by ruptured capillaries leaking blood into the tissues which form the skin.

This bleeding causes the characteristic purple, black and blue skin discolouration. This may also be accompanied by tenderness and pain. The discolouration gradually reduces, with the colour becoming green or yellow before completely resolving in around 2 weeks.

Haematomas
Usually caused by blunt trauma, a haematoma is a confined collection of clotted blood.

Most haematomas heal uneventfully; however, some may require treatment to prevent long-term disfigurement and resulting scar tissue, particularly those involving the face and head. Patients may be advised to regularly massage the affected area to help break down the clot and hopefully prevent the formation of scar tissue. Prompt treatment may be required for those haematomas involving the ear or nose. Treatment would involve incision and drainage of the haematoma followed by a compression dressing. Untreated ear haematomas may lead to disfigurement of the ear resulting from the collected clotted blood separating the cartilage from other tissues and vessels. In untreated cases this tissue separation causes the cartilage to die. This results in the area becoming pale and shrivelled. In addition to this fibrous scar tissue also forms over time, resulting in the characteristic 'cauliflower ear' (a condition which frequently affects boxers and rugby players).

TEMPROMANDIBULAR JOINT DISORDER (TMJD)

This term is used to describe a dysfunction of the temporomandibular joint (TMJ) and its associated muscles. Rather than arthritis, TMJD is usually a

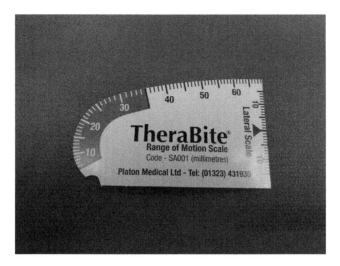

Figure 7.5 TheraBite range of motion scale.

muscular condition caused by overloading the muscles of mastication. In the majority of cases, TMJD responds well to conservative treatment. For some individuals the symptoms of TMJD can be painful and distressing, resulting in a negative impact on their quality of life. The symptoms of TMJD can include crepitus which is a clicking, grating or popping noise from the joint area caused by the cartilage disc within the joint moving slightly out of position. Symptoms may also include chronic pain, limited mouth opening and the feeling that the joint is locked.

During the patient's assessment, consent and a detailed history of the symptoms will be taken followed by an intra- and extra-oral examination. The maxillofacial surgeon will usually palpate the joint area and associated muscles while asking the patient to open and close their mouth. The clinician may also utilise a disposable paper range-of-motion scale (Figure 7.5) to accurately measure the patient's mouth opening. Should it be necessary, medical imagining of the TMJ (Figure 7.6) may be requested.

Conservative treatment

Patients should be reassured that symptoms of TMJD usually respond well to joint rest, conservative treatment and lifestyle changes. Advice given may include:

- Avoid wide mouth opening such as yawning or when eating.
- Soft diet: refrain from hard or chewy foods.
- Be aware of and avoid parafunction habits, for example nail biting and pen chewing.

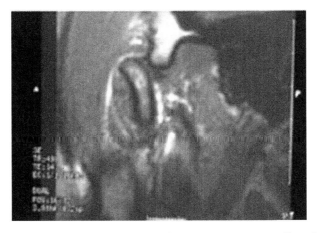

Figure 7.6 Temporomandibular joint. Source: Pedro Diz Dios, Crispian Scully, Oslei Paes de Almeida, Jose V. Bagán, Adalberto Mosqueda Taylor, 2016. *Oral Medicine and Pathology at a Glance*, 2nd Edition, p. 96. Reproduced with permission of John Wiley & Sons.

- Grinding and clenching, particularly during sleep, can cause significant TMJD symptoms and may be an indication of stress in the individual's life which may need to be addressed.
- Gentle tongue and jaw exercises performed regularly as directed by the clinician.
- The application of gentle heat to the affected area, such as a warm water bottle or heated, folded towel.
- The use of paracetamol and non-steroidal anti-inflammatory drugs (NSAIDs) under the direction of the clinician may also be recommended.

A small number of patients may require further investigation or treatment such as arthrocentesis or arthroscopy.

Arthrocentesis

Arthrocentesis is a surgical procedure in which sterile fluid is used to wash out the TMJ with an aim of returning the cartilage disc to the correct position and removing any debris from inside the joint. Arthrocentesis is performed while the patient is asleep under general anaesthetic. Local anaesthetic is administered to the TMJ site and two needles are inserted in front of the ear into the joint. Sterile fluid is passed under pressure through one needle and allowed to flow out of the second. During the procedure, the maxillofacial surgeon may manipulate the patient's jaw in an attempt to realign the cartilage disc. At the end of the procedure the surgeon may administer a steroid drug directly into the joint. Arthrocentesis can also be performed during an arthroscopic examination.

Arthroscopy

An arthroscope is used to examine inside joints and is used for diagnostic and sometimes surgical procedures such as removal of scar tissue. It is a small camera/telescope that projects an imagine onto a connected monitor. Arthroscopies are sometimes referred to as keyhole surgery. As with arthrocentesis, it is performed with the patient under a general anaesthetic. Following the administration of local anaesthetic, a small incision is made in front of the ear. The arthroscope is inserted through the incision into the jaw joint. Should the maxillofacial surgeon require other instruments, a second incision is made to facilitate their use.

SALIVARY GLAND SURGERY

A patient who presents with an unexplained swelling or lump relating to a salivary gland will be referred to a maxillofacial surgeon for investigation.

Sialolithiasis

Also known as salivary calculi or salivary stones, sialolithiasis (Figure 7.7) are calcified masses which form in the salivary glands and ducts. They can vary in size from a few millimetres to several centimetres. Usually affecting the submandibular duct, the calculi can cause either a partial or complete obstruction of the duct. Symptoms may include a history of recurrent pain and swelling, particularly when salivary flow is stimulated at mealtimes, a lump intra-orally in

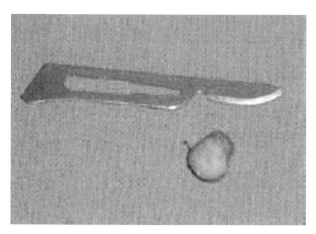

Figure 7.7 Sialolithiasis. Source: Pedro Diz Dios, Crispian Scully, Oslei Paes de Almeida, Jose V. Bagán, Adalberto Mosqueda Taylor, 2016. *Oral Medicine and Pathology at a Glance*, 2nd Edition, p.78. Reproduced with permission of John Wiley & Sons.

the region of a salivary duct, and also hyposalivation. Diagnosis of sialolithiasis may require radiographic examination. Calculi affecting the submandibular duct may be visible on plain film radiographs. Should the suspected stone not be visible, then imagining by sialogram may be requested. CT or MRI scans may also be considered.

Sialogram

A sialogram (Figure 7.8) is a type of radiograph which uses a contrast dye to aid diagnosis of sialolithiasis and other possible salivary conditions. Prior to the radiograph a cannula is inserted into the identified duct and a contrast medium is injected via the cannula into the duct. The dye will aid the visibility of the duct on the produced image.

Treatment

Some small salivary calculi may resolve spontaneously if the stone passes out of the duct and into the mouth. However, removal of larger stones is frequently necessary. If upon examination the position of the stone within the duct is identifiable, surgical removal may be performed under local anaesthesia. This would involve a small incision in the area of the stone. Once the stone has been successfully removed, the incision may be left unsutured to heal. Other methods of removal may require an endoscopic procedure known as a sialendoscopy.

Sialendoscopy

A small endoscope is inserted through the identified duct towards the salivary gland. This procedure may be performed under either local or general anaesthesia. Sialendoscopy may be used for diagnosis or therapeutic treatment.

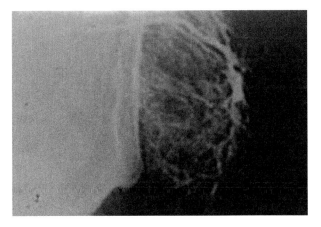

Figure 7.8 Sialogram in sialolithiasis. Source: Pedro Diz Dios, Crispian Scully, Oslei Paes de Almeida, Jose V. Bagán, Adalberto Mosqueda Taylor, 2016. *Oral Medicine and Pathology at a Glance*, 2nd Edition, p. 10. Reproduced with permission of John Wiley & Sons.

TRAUMA AND COMPLEX PROCEDURES

Instruments can be passed through the endoscope to treat blockages to the duct and remove calculi.

Parotidectomy

Parotidectomy is a surgical procedure to remove all or part of the parotid gland. During this procedure, an incision is made in front of the ear extending down into the neck. A flap is then raised to expose the parotid gland. The facial nerve runs through the gland and needs to identified and protected in an attempt to prevent its damage. In some cases the facial nerve may become damaged; if it forms part of the malignancy, it may need to be removed. An attempt to repair branches of the facial nerve which have been divided may be made with grafts from the great auricular nerve. Permanent facial weakness and palsy may result from damage to the facial nerve. In all cases, the earlobe is likely to remain numb after other areas have recovered.

Tumours affecting the salivary glands

- **Benign tumours:** The majority of salivary gland tumours are benign including pleomorphic adenomas and Warthin's tumour. The most common of these is pleomorphic adenoma. This tumour is a low-grade, slow-growing tumour.
- **Malignant tumours:** There are several types of malignancy, some of which are very rare, which can affect the salivary glands. The majority of malignant tumours develop in the parotid gland. The main groups of malignant tumour are mucoepidermoid carcinoma, adenoidcystic carcinoma and adenocarcinoma.
- **Mucoepidermoid carcinoma:** This is a cancer of the cells which line the salivary gland. It forms as small cysts. It is usually low grade and slow growing, although it can be high grade. Mucoepidermoid tumours usually develop in the parotid gland; however, they can on occasion develop in the submandibular and minor salivary glands.
- **Adenoidcystic tumours:** These types of tumours are uncommon. They present in the mouth or on the face as a painless slow-growing mass.
- **Actinic cell adenocarcinoma:** This type of tumour is usually slow growing and is most likely to affect the parotid gland.

    The maxillofacial surgeon may arrange for diagnosis of the presenting mass by biopsy and fine needle aspiration, therefore allowing for a histology report. Medical scans may also be requested at this time. These investigations are described further in Chapter 6.

TRAUMA AND COMPLEX PROCEDURES

CRANIOFACIAL AND ORAL CANCER

Cancer is when specific cells reproduce abnormally and uncontrollably. These abnormal cells can, in some instances, spread to surrounding healthy organs and tissue. The type of cancer which can spread is referred to as malignant. Not all cancers spread. This type of non- malignant tumour is known as benign. Maxillofacial surgeons diagnose and treat cancer of the head, neck and mouth. This includes cancer involving the skin, salivary glands, oral cavity and oropharynx. Areas of the oral cavity include:

- Lips.
- The gingiva and mucosa.
- Floor of the mouth.
- The hard palate.
- Anterior two-thirds of the tongue.

    Areas of the oropharynx include:

- The posterior third of the tongue.
- The soft palate.
- The tonsils.
- The posterior wall of the throat.

    There are definite risk factors which increase the chance of developing cancer of these structures. Smoking and alcohol consumption are the main risk factors for cancer of the oral cavity and oropharynx. Exposure to ultraviolet light (UV) through sunlight or by using sun beds is the main risk factor for cancer involving the skin of the face and neck. Human papilloma virus (HPV) has also been linked to some cancers of the oral and oropharyngeal areas. HPV usually causes no harm, resolving without any treatment. However, some sexual activities may increase the risk of a person developing HPV-related cancer; the risk increases with the number of sexual partners an individual has.

Types of oral cancer

Dysplasia

During a histopathology examination, cells are studied microscopically. Normal cells go through changes prior to becoming cancerous. Cells which look abnormal but are not yet cancerous are described as dysplasia. These cells may or may not become cancerous, but do show underlying changes.

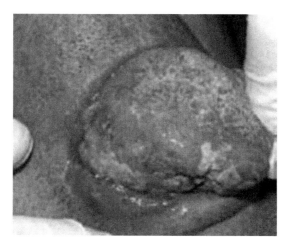

Figure 7.9 Squamous cell carcinoma. Source: Pedro Diz Dios, Crispian Scully, Oslei Paes de Almeida, Jose V. Bagán, Adalberto Mosqueda Taylor, 2016. *Oral Medicine and Pathology at a Glance*, 2nd Edition, p. 50. Reproduced with permission of John Wiley & Sons.

Squamous cell carcinoma (SCC)

A total of 90% of all oral cancer is squamous cell carcinoma (Figure 7.9). Squamous cells are flat cells found in the outer part of the epidermis, oral mucosa, lips, tongue and several other areas of the body.

Basal cell carcinoma

Basal cells are epithelial cells found in the deepest area of the skin. Basal cell cancers are linked to sun exposure and UV light from sun beds. Common areas affected are the face, head, neck and ears. Basal cell carcinomas are usually localised; however, they can invade deeply. These lesions are usually painless and slow growing. Their presentation can be varied, ranging from a small, pearly, translucent and raised area which may have noticeable blood vessels to a lesion which is sunken and crusty and which bleeds easily if knocked. Basal cell carcinoma's are sometimes referred to as 'rodent ulcers'.

Melanoma

This type of cancer (Figure 7.10) affects the melanocyte cells which give colour and pigment to tissues, including the skin. There are several sub-types of melanoma, but the most common is superficial spreading melanoma. The main risk factor in developing melanoma is exposure to UV light, with fair-skinned people and individuals with moles being more at risk.

Lymphoma

Oral lymphoma (Figure 7.11) can manifest anywhere within the oral cavity. It starts as a non-specific swelling. The cause of non-Hodgkin lymphoma is

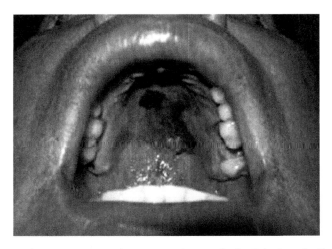

Figure 7.10 Melanoma. Source: Pedro Diz Dios, Crispian Scully, Oslei Paes de Almeida, Jose V. Bagán, Adalberto Mosqueda Taylor, 2016. *Oral Medicine and Pathology at a Glance*, 2nd Edition, p. 32. Reproduced with permission of John Wiley & Sons.

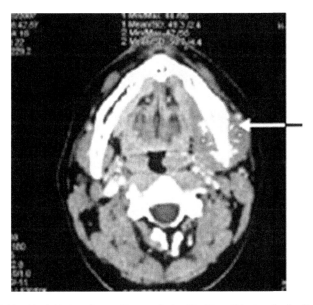

Figure 7.11 Non-Hodgkin lymphoma. Source: Pedro Diz Dios, Crispian Scully, Oslei Paes de Almeida, Jose V. Bagán, Adalberto Mosqueda Taylor, 2016. *Oral Medicine and Pathology at a Glance*, 2nd Edition, p. 52. Reproduced with permission of John Wiley & Sons.

not clear, but maxillofacial surgeons and dentists can aid its early diagnosis and therefore play a vital role when undertaking an extra oral examination. Non-Hodgkin lymphoma is a cancer that starts in the lymph nodes, spreading to other areas of the body via the blood vessels and lymphatic system.

TRAUMA AND COMPLEX PROCEDURES

The lymph nodes are not painful, despite being enlarged. The enlargement is not associated with the lymph node but lymphoid ectopic (occurs in an area that is not its customary environment) tissue. The most common lymph nodes affected are those in the neck since they are numerous in this area; however, other lymph nodes within the body can also be affected. Other symptoms of this condition are night sweats, fevers and typically weight loss. Once diagnosed, the treatment for non-Hodgkin lymphoma normally encompasses chemo- and radiotherapy.

Referral and diagnosis

Clinicians referring patients with what they believe to be possible cancer use specific suspected cancer pathway referral systems. The aim of such pathways is to allow patients with suspected cancer to see a specialist within 2 weeks from referral. As discussed in Chapter 4, a detailed initial assessment and clinical examination of the patient will be performed by the maxillofacial consultant. Should the consultant believe that the lesion is suspicious, then urgent investigations will be performed. These may include investigatory procedures such as histological biopsy and fine needle aspiration (FNA). Medical imaging including ultrasound, computerised tomography (CT) and magnetic resonance imaging (MRI) scan may be ordered (Figure 7.11). These procedures and scans are described in Chapter 6. The reports from the investigations and imagery will provide the maxillofacial surgeon with the information he/she needs to give a diagnosis and stage the cancer.

TNM staging

Cancer of the oral cavity and oropharynx is staged using a T (tumour) – N (nodes) – M (metastasis) system.

T refers to the size of the primary tumour:

- **T1:** the tumour is not larger than 2 cm.
- **T2:** the tumour is of size 2–4 cm.
- **T3:** the tumour is larger than 4 cm.
- **T4a:** the tumour has invaded nearby body tissues such as the skin, bone, tongue or sinuses.
- **T4b:** the tumour has spread into surrounding structures such as around the jaws, the base of the skull and the carotid arteries.

N refers to whether the cancer has spread into the lymph nodes or not:

- **N0:** no cancer cells in the lymph nodes.
- **N1:** cancer cells are present in one lymph node (less than 3 cm) on the same side of the neck as the cancer.

- **N2a:** cancer cells are present in one lymph node (of size 3–6 cm) on the same side of the neck as the cancer.
- **N2b:** cancer cells are present in more than one lymph node (less than 6 cm) on the same side of the neck as the cancer.
- **N2c:** cancer cells are present in nodes (less than 6 cm) on the other side of the neck and/or both sides to the cancer.
- **N3:** cancer cells are present in at least one lymph node (more than 6 cm).

M refers to whether the cancer has spread to other areas of the body or not.

- **M0:** the cancer has not spread to other areas of the body.
- **M1:** the cancer has spread to other areas of the body.

The overall TNM score would, for example, be displayed as T2, N1, M0. This would indicate that the tumour is of size 2–4 cm, cancer cells are in present in one lymph node (less than 3 cm) on the same side of the neck as the tumour and that the cancer has not spread to other areas of the body.

The multidisciplinary team

Cancer treatment is planned by a group of surgeons, clinicians and healthcare professionals known as a multidisciplinary team (MDT). The role of the MDT is to meet regularly to recommend and plan the best treatment based on:

- The patient's general health.
- The type of cancer and its stage.
- Recommended pathways and treatments.

The MDT may include:

- Consultant surgeons (maxillofacial, ENT and plastic surgeons).
- Consultant oncologists.
- Consultant radiologists.
- Consultant pathologists.
- Consultant restorative dentists.
- Maxillofacial technicians.
- Specialist head and neck nurses.
- Dieticians.
- Speech and language therapists.
- Physiotherapists.
- Macmillan nurses.

The MDT will discuss each patient's case regularly. Cancer treatments such as surgery, radiotherapy and chemotherapy will be planned during these meetings. The planned treatment will then need to be discussed in detail with the patient for them to be able to give consent for treatment to commence. Should

TRAUMA AND COMPLEX PROCEDURES

the treatment plan be altered at any point, the patient must be fully advised and consent for the new treatment plan gained.

Treatment of oral cancer

Radical (comprehensive) neck dissection

This is a planned surgical procedure which is usually performed at the same time as surgery to remove the tumour. A radical neck dissection is performed when there is evidence that several lymph nodes are affected. The aim of this dissection is to remove the lymph nodes. An incision is made which extends in a Y-shape from behind the ear and under the chin down into the neck. All lymph nodes are sent for histology reporting.

Selective (partial) neck dissection

Should there be a suspicion that only a small amount of cancer cells are present in the nodes of the neck, then a partial dissection is performed. In the case of a selective neck dissection, only nodes which are most likely to be affected by the patient's type of cancer are removed for further investigation.

Surgery

Surgery involves not only removal of the tumour, but also reconstruction of the affected area in order to repair defects caused by the tumour and its removal. The aim of reconstruction is to reproduce function and appearance by replacing the lost tissue. There are various methods of reconstruction, all of which have advantages and disadvantages.

Radial forearm free flap

This is a frequently used method of free tissue transfer. It can be used to reconstruct large areas of the head, neck and mouth. It is particularly useful when reconstructing areas of the mouth as the tissue does not shrink during healing, hopefully reducing the degree to which speech and swallowing is affected. Tissue is removed from the patient's inner forearm. The tissue removed includes skin and fat along with the artery and vein vessels. Once successfully removed, the tissue flap is placed in the area to be reconstructed. The blood vessels (artery and vein) are connected to nearby vessels to enable the flap to remain vital while it heals.

The forearm is then also reconstructed with borrowed tissue from another area.

Fibula free flap

The fibula is the smaller bone found in the lower leg. It is a small thin bone that can be entirely removed without affecting the ability to bear weight. As with all free flaps, the bone is removed along with the artery and vein vessels.

TRAUMA AND COMPLEX PROCEDURES

Once the bone is transferred to the area in need of reconstruction, these blood vessels are connected to vessels in the neck. The harvested bone is then secured into position with small plates and screws.

Temporalis flap

A temporalis flap differs from a free flap as it remains attached to its blood supply throughout its repositioning. Following an incision, the temporalis muscle is carefully raised from the skull. Once successfully raised, the muscle is tunnelled into the oral cavity to repair the defect.

Nasolabial flap

Similar to the temporalis flap, the nasolabial flap utilises the nasolabial tissue folds. These folds are the lines which run along both sides of the nose down towards the corners of the mouth. Following an incision along the nasolabial line, the surgeon raises a flap which remains attached to its blood supply throughout. This flap can be performed unilaterally or bilaterally. Areas which can be reconstructed in this way include repairs to the anterior floor of the mouth. The raised flap would be tunnelled into the mouth where it would be placed to reconstruct the area.

There are occasions when a flap cannot be used to reconstruct an area. An obturator is a removable prosthesis designed to repair the defect. They are constructed by specialist maxillofacial technicians.

Radiotherapy
External beam radiotherapy

Radiotherapy uses radiation to kill cancer cells. Radiotherapy may be used as a primary treatment of cancer. However, in many cases it is used as an adjuvant treatment following surgery. It may also be used in palliative care to relieve symptoms in those who are terminally ill. Radiotherapy is usually delivered by an external beam from a machine which is similar to that of an X-ray machine. A course of treatment is planned and usually requires the patient to have multiple exposures over a series of weeks. Patients undergoing radiotherapy are required to remain very still during active exposure. Markers or specially made patient masks may be used to ensure that the patient remains still and that the radiation is carefully targeted to the required area.

Internal radiotherapy

Occasionally internal radiotherapy is used; this is known as brachytherapy. Brachytherapy involves a source of radiation being directly implanted into the tumour which then stays *in situ* for a prescribed number of days.

Side-effects

Radiotherapy has side-effects. All radiotherapy causes general side-effects including tiredness and red, sore skin at the exposure site. However, radiotherapy to the head and neck area can cause other side-effects including: a sore mouth and throat; difficulties with swallowing; dry mouth; taste and smell disturbances; and difficulties with mouth opening.

Chemotherapy

Chemotherapy uses drugs to disrupt the growth of cancer cells and destroy them. Chemotherapy may be used if the cancer needs to be shrunk before any surgery can be performed to remove the tumour; this is referred to as neoadjuvant chemotherapy. As with radiotherapy, chemotherapy may be used as part of a palliative care plan. This may be the case if a cancer has returned after previous surgery and radiotherapy treatment. The chemotherapy would be used to control the growth of the tumour in order to relieve symptoms.

Chemotherapy has unpleasant side-effects, including: hair loss; vomiting; diarrhoea; tiredness; mouth ulcers; and blood cell changes.

Chemotherapy and radiotherapy

In some cases, chemotherapy and radiotherapy may be used at the same time. This is known as chemoradiation. The chemotherapy drugs can in some instances help the radiotherapy to be more effective. This treatment is intense, and patients undergoing chemoradiation therapy experience unpleasant side-effects from both the radiation and medication.

CLEFT LIP AND PALATE

As the lip and the palate develop separately, it is possible for a cleft lip (Figure 7.12) to occur without a cleft palate; likewise, a cleft palate can occur without a cleft lip, or they can occur together. Cleft lip and cleft palate can also occur on one or both sides (Figure 7.13) of the mouth.

When the palate forms it is initially in two halves. When these two halves do not fuse naturally, clefts occur. The two halves of the palate start to fuse approximately 8 weeks after conception. Clefts can be either complete or partial and may only involve the soft palate or the hard and soft palate (Figure 7.14). A complete cleft lip and palate is a result of failure of the gingiva and the lip to join together. Occasionally the gingiva may not be affected as the gingiva and the lip start to fuse, but the process is not completed. This process starts approximately 6 weeks after conception.

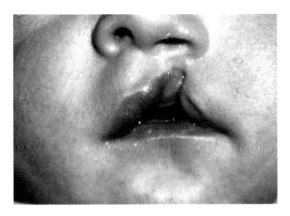

Figure 7.12 Cleft lip. Source: Grist, F. 2010. *Basic Guide to Orthodontic Dental Nursing.*
Reproduced with permission of John Wiley & Sons.

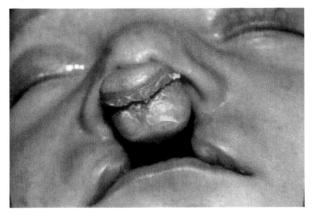

Figure 7.13 Bilateral left. Source: Grist, F. 2010. *Basic Guide to Orthodontic Dental Nursing.*
Reproduced with permission of John Wiley & Sons.

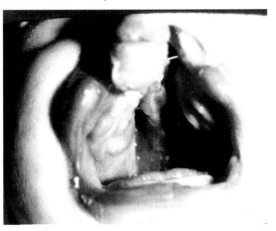

Figure 7.14 Cleft of the lip, hard and soft plates. Source: Grist, F. 2010. *Basic Guide to
Orthodontic Dental Nursing.* Reproduced with permission of John Wiley & Sons.

TRAUMA AND COMPLEX PROCEDURES

Children born with a cleft lip may suffer physical and psychological effects such as speech and hearing problems, resulting in difficulties communicating and lack of confidence. These could have further consequences later in life.

The causes of clefts are not fully known. It is thought that a combination of genetic and other factors attribute to their occurrence. Risk factors during pregnancy could include: a lack of folic acid if the mother consumed alcohol and/or smoked; a poor nutritional diet; obesity of the pregnant mother; or whether certain medications were taken.

Cleft lip or cleft palate are easy to diagnose. They can be detected during prenatal ultrasounds or once the baby has been born through a physical examination of the mouth, nose and palate. Once a cleft lip and palate have been diagnosed, patients are referred to an NHS specialist unit where they are treated by a multidisciplinary team that comprises:

- Surgeon.
- Paediatrician.
- Ear, nose and throat surgeon.
- Orthodontist.
- Hygienist.
- Psychologist.
- Speech and language therapist.
- Specialist dental nurses.
- Specialist cleft registered general nurses.
- Audiologist.

Most patients receive a similar care plan that commences as soon as the baby is born to aid feeding, and concludes at the age of 15 under the care of the orthodontist. During this time, patients receive surgery to correct the cleft lip and palate and receive speech therapy. Following this, patients attend outpatient clinics for regular reviews and appropriate treatment as required. To monitor the patient's progress, records are made of the patient's development at the age of 5, 10, 15 and 20.

For some children, correction of a cleft lip and palate can involve many operations and stays in hospital; this can impact on the children and their parents or carers, as it stressful and traumatic for all. For other children, good results can be achieved following a few operations. Children with cleft lips and palates will require intervention from other specialist services such as a dentist, speech therapist and audiologist.

Surgery to repair a cleft lip is undertaken when the child is approximately 3 months old. The corrective surgery is undertaken with a general anaesthetic, and the procedure normally takes 1–2 hours or longer if the cleft is more extensive. It involves the cleft lip being repaired along with the underlying muscles, with the nose invariably being restructured at the same time. As the child will

TRAUMA AND COMPLEX PROCEDURES

be left with a slight scar, the surgeon will endeavour to line the scar up with any natural lines of the lip.

Surgery to repair the palate is undertaken when the child is aged 6–12 months. This corrective surgery is also undertaken using a general anaesthetic, and the procedure takes approximately 2 hours. It involves rearrangement of the lining of the palate along with the muscles; no extra tissue is normally required to complete this operation. Some patients, as previously explained, may require further surgery for the following reasons:

- To improve the appearance and function of the lips and palate.
- A hole may appear in the palate early on during the healing phase, which requires repair.
- The palate is not functioning properly during speech.
- If there is a cleft in the gingiva a bone graft operation is required to repair the alveolar cleft. This will be undertaken when the child is approximately 9–12 years old.
- If the growth patterns of the jaws are unequal.

BISPHOSPHONATE-RELATED OSTEONECROSIS OF THE JAW (BRONJ)

Bisphosphonate-related osteonecrosis of the jaw (Figure 7.15) is an area of exposed or dead bone that has been present for more than two months in an individual who has received, or is currently receiving, bisphosphonate therapy. These patients have usually undergone an invasive dental treatment such as an extraction. Bisphosphonates are a group of drugs used to treat osteoporosis and diseases of the bone, such as some cancers. They are administered either orally or intravenously.

Although the risk of developing bisphosphonate-related osteonecrosis is low, it is thought that the risk is increased when administered by intravenous infusion. To mitigate this risk, any patient with a history of bisphosphonate treatment should receive prophylactic and local measures when having oral surgery, including simple extractions.

Many maxillofacial departments use agreed algorithms to determine which of the following prophylactic and local measures an individual requires; these may include:

- Detailed medical history (including the presence of any co-morbidities).
- Pre-surgical chlorhexidine mouthwash.
- Haemostatic dressing.
- Sutures.
- Prescribed post-surgical chlorhexidine mouthwash.

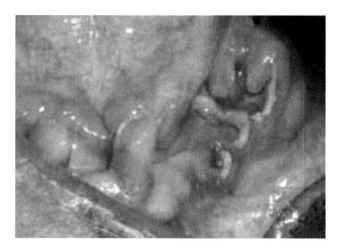

Figure 7.15 Bisphosphonate-related osteonecrosis. Source: Pedro Diz Dios, Crispian Scully, Oslei Paes de Almeida, Jose V. Bagán, Adalberto Mosqueda Taylor, 2016. *Oral Medicine and Pathology at a Glance*, 2nd Edition, p. 52. Reproduced with permission of John Wiley & Sons.

- Antibiotic prophylaxis.
- A review appointment.
- Excellent post-extraction/surgery advice and instruction.

ANTICOAGULANT AND ANTIPLATELET MEDICATION

Anticoagulant or antiplatelet medicines inhibit blood clotting. They are prescribed to patients in high-risk groups in order to prevent the development of blood clots which may lead to serious conditions such as stroke, deep vein thrombosis and heart attack.

Warfarin and newer anticoagulants such as Rivaroxaban interrupt the clotting cascade by inhibiting the complex factors need for coagulation. Patients taking warfarin require careful monitoring of their international normalised ratio (INR). This is normally undertaken at the patient's doctor's surgery or within an outpatient department (Figure 7.16). The patient will carry a warning card which contains information relating to their current INR status. An INR scale 1 is normal, that is, no anticoagulant medication with clotting time being approximately 3–5 minutes. An INR of 2 indicates that it will take twice the normal time to achieve coagulation, and so on. A patient's target INR is set according to their medical history. Dependent upon the maxillofacial surgery being performed, the maxillofacial surgeon will require evidence of the patient's current INR status. Provided this is at an acceptable level for the planned procedure and the patient has not had any sickness or diarrhoea,

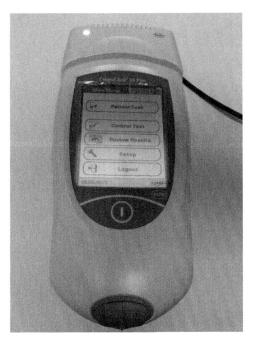

Figure 7.16 Roche CoaguChek XS Plus.

then treatment proceeds. If this is not the case, the maxillofacial surgeon will request an INR test. The outcome of this test will decide whether the patient receives treatment, or is rebooked until the INR count is at an acceptable level to reflect the treatment in hand. Diet can affect the patient's INR, particularly food high in Vitamin K. It is therefore advisable that a stable diet is maintained.

Antiplatelet drugs work in a different way to anticoagulants. Clopidogrel and also low-dose aspirin (acetylsalicylic acid) inhibit the ability of the platelets to stick together to form a clot.

As part of an assessment appointment, the maxillofacial surgeon will discuss the prescribed medication and any impact it will have on treatment, and advise the patient accordingly. During surgical procedures, either of these forms of treatments may, by their nature, extend the length of haemorrhage prior to a clot forming. In advance of a surgical procedure, a patient taking warfarin will require a current INR reading to ensure that it is safe to proceed.

Following any surgical intervention to ensure successful haemostasis, local measures such as haemostatic agents and sutures may be utilised. The patient would need to be provided with comprehensive verbal and written post-operative instructions, with specific advice regarding their medication and the possibility of further haemorrhage. It would also be prudent to warn

TRAUMA AND COMPLEX PROCEDURES

the patient that, due to the effect of their medication, they may experience more bruising than usual.

ORTHOGNATHIC SURGERY

Orthognathic surgery is a multidisciplinary area involving specialists from both maxillofacial surgery and orthodontics departments. Orthognathic directly translates as 'straight jaws'. This type of treatment combines both orthodontic treatment with surgical intervention and is used to correct jaw discrepancies, such as position and size, and severe malocclusion where orthodontic treatment alone would be insufficient. These discrepancies can impact an individual's quality of life, affecting their facial appearance, jaw function and speech.

Referral to a hospital outpatients department for an initial specialist assessment is usually made by the patient's dentist or orthodontist. The patient is usually seen by a consultant orthodontist in a joint clinic with a consultant maxillofacial surgeon. The purpose of this first assessment appointment is to discuss with the patient the suitability of surgery and the possible, expected outcome from the treatment.

During such an initial assessment, intra- and extra-oral and radiographic examinations are performed. These radiographs may include dental panoramic tomography and lateral cephalometric images. The patient's medical and social history is also noted, along with a discussion relating to their personal views regarding the reason for the referral. Study models and photographs may also be taken to accurately record the patient's current presentation. If indicated, both the orthodontist and the maxillofacial surgeon will explain to the patient the treatment process and surgery involved following the process for informed consent.

As orthognathic surgery is only suitable once an individual is no longer actively growing, those patients under the age of 18 are usually kept under review by the specialists until such time that facial growth has ceased. Following assessment, orthognathic treatment is split into four clearly defined areas:

- Pre-surgical phase.
- Surgery.
- Post-surgical phase.
- Retention.

Prior to any treatment, if the patient has third molars teeth present (erupted or unerupted) these will need extracting as the position of the third molars impedes the proposed orthognathic surgical site. Once this is completed, the pre-surgical phase of fixed appliance treatment can commence, which may last

12–18 months. Once this pre-surgical orthodontic phase is complete, detailed measurements are taken and the orthodontist will arrange for an occlusal wafer to be constructed. This wafer is an acrylic occlusion guide for the maxillofacial surgeon to use during surgery. Orthognathic surgical procedures are referred to as osteotomies. Osteotomies may involve just the maxilla or mandible. In some cases however, osteotomies are bimaxillary, involving both the maxilla and mandible.

Maxillary osteotomies

Osteotomies of the maxilla may be at Le Fort I, Le Fort II or Le fort III levels (Figure 7.2). Le Fort I is the most common (see 'Fractures of the mid-face' earlier in this chapter). Surgery for the Le Fort I osteotomy is carried out from inside the mouth so that there are no visible scars. An incision is made through the gingiva above the upper teeth. The tissue is then retracted to gain access to the underlying bone. The maxilla is then cut with a small saw to allow it to be broken in a controlled manner. It is then guided into its new position with the occlusal wafer and held with a form of inter-maxillary fixation (IMF) such as elastics. Once it is correctly positioned, small surgical metal plates and screws are placed to hold the new position. The occlusion is then checked and the incision is then closed with absorbable sutures.

Mandibular osteotomies

The surgical procedure for a sagittal split osteotomy is performed from inside the mouth so that there are no visible scars. However, small incisions are very occasionally required.

An incision is made through the gingiva behind the lower molars. The tissues are then retracted to gain access to the mandible. The inner cortical plate of the ramus is cut horizontally. The outer plate is cut vertically in line with the second molar region. These two cuts are then joined by a third cut, which joins them all together. This is then repeated on the other side of the mandible. Once this is completed, the mandible is split along these cut lines. In an attempt to prevent permanent loss of feeling, the maxillofacial surgeon will endeavour to preserve the inferior dental nerve and other vessels which run inside the mandible. The mandible is then guided into its new position with the occlusal wafer and held in place with a form of IMF. Once it is correctly positioned, small surgical metal plates and screws are placed to hold the new position. The occlusion is then checked and the incisions are closed with absorbable sutures. Wound drainage may be required immediately after surgery to prevent excess swelling and bruising. Patients will remain in hospital for 1–2 nights until the maxillofacial surgeon believes they are ready to be discharged. Post-surgery radiographs are taken to check jaw position before discharge. While the new occlusion is

TRAUMA AND COMPLEX PROCEDURES

settling, IMF by elastics is usually needed. The orthodontist will adjust the pattern of these elastics during the post-surgical appointments in the outpatient's department. Once the occlusion is well established and healing complete, the post-surgical phase is completed as planned. Follow-up appointments with the maxillofacial surgeon are also arranged to check on healing and provide advice regarding any post-operative problems.

DENTAL IMPLANTS

A dental implant is a titanium root-sized prosthesis introduced into healthy bone to supply a firm anchor in the mandible/maxilla, to which is attached either dentures or a crown.

Many patients have dental implants to replace missing teeth as opposed to partial dentures and bridges. Other reasons for them being placed are to support a bridge to prevent putting a healthy tooth at risk by preparing it as an abutment, to aid the retention of existing dentures and to repair a jawbone that has resorbed due to the loss of teeth. For patients to have dental implants inserted they must have strong jaw bones, healthy gingiva and general good dental health. If a patient smokes a dental implant is likely to fail as their dental health is generally poor. The success rate of dental implants is high providing the patient has a good oral hygiene regime. A patient must undergo a proper consultation with a dental implantologist to allow them to assess the patient's suitability for dental implants. This will involve intra-oral and extra-oral examinations to evaluate the state of the patient's jaws and teeth. X-rays will be taken to look at the condition of the bone and impressions taken to make sure the implants being made match the shape and size of the existing teeth. Naturally, the implantologist will provide the patient with an explanation of the procedure along with making the patient aware of the commitment required by them. Consent and medical history will be taken.

Procedure

During the first stage, the patient is settled in the dental chair and provided with personal protective equipment. The implantologist will re-check the status of their medical history and ensure consent is in place and still valid. A brief explanation of the procedure is provided. For pain and anxiety control, topical anaesthetic might be placed prior to the administration of the local anaesthetic. Quite often patients have intravenous sedation when having dental implants, as the appointment is lengthy and deemed an unusual procedure.

The patient is given 5 mL mouthwash of chlorhexidine gluconate to swill around their mouth for a few minutes. The patient is constantly monitored and reassured. The nurse assisting with the dental implants will wash their

TRAUMA AND COMPLEX PROCEDURES

hands using the recognised method and gown up for the surgical procedure, assisted by the circulation nurse. The patient is then prepared by the scrub nurse who drapes the patient from head to toe to maintain a sterile field. The implantologist, who is also assisted by the circulation nurse, will scrub and gown up in the same manner as the dental nurse.

The implantologist will check the area anaesthetised to ensure it is numb. An incision in the gingiva where the dental implants are to be placed is made with a No. 15 Bard-Parker scalpel blade. A gingival flap is raised using either a Mitchell's trimmer or a Howarth's periosteal elevator. The flap is retracted with an Austin's tissue retractor to aid visibility and make it easier for the maxillofacial surgeon to use the straight surgical hand-piece. A straight surgical hand-piece with an irrigation tube containing 0.9% sodium chloride solution, attached to a small rosehead surgical bur, is used to make a small hole in the jaw. The size of the bur will depend upon the size of the implant and the system being used.

Once the correct size has been prepared, a titanium implant is inserted where it will bond to the bone, known as osseointegration. A closure screw is paced on top of the titanium post. As healing takes time, the patient will require a further appointment to have the bridge or denture attached to the dental implant. The implantologist will therefore suture the flap back into place using Kilner needle holders, an absorbable suture, Gillie's tissue dissecting forceps, a Kilner cheek retractor and long pointed scissors.

If the patient received intravenous sedation they will be recovered, assessed for discharge, issued with post-operative care instructions and permitted to leave the dental surgery with their escort. If the patient only received a local anaesthetic, they will be given post-operative care instructions. Whichever form of pain and anxiety control used, the patient will be provided with a further appointment for the second stage. During the healing stage, the patient will see the implantologist on a regular basis so they can assess if the implant is still firmly attached prior to the denture or bridge being placed. The patient must ensure they maintain good oral health to avoid rejection, and can experience swelling and pain where the dental implants have been placed.

During the second stage, once the bone and jaws have been allowed to heal and the dental implant is secure, the denture or bridge is firmly attached to the implant.

TONGUE-TIE RELEASE

Frenectomy

A frenectomy, which involves the removal of a frenulum, is also known as a frenulectomy. A frenulum is a band of fibrous tissue covered with mucous membrane. The reason for their removal is that they restrict the movement of an organ within the body. Within the mouth there are two frenulums:

- **The lingual frenulum:** This is present in the mouth under the tongue and is attached to the floor of the mouth.
- **The labial frenulum:** This is present in the mouth under the upper lip and is attached to the gingiva above the central incisors.

Lingual frenulum

A lingual frenulum is removed due to patients suffering from ankyloglossia. This is commonly referred to as tongue-tied. A patient who suffers from this condition will have an abnormally short, thick frenulum with some patients having their tongue completely bound to the floor of the mouth. This can not only have an effect on their lives socially, due to limited movement, but will also affect their oral hygiene, eating and speech.

Labial frenulum

A labial frenulum is removed when it is attached to the centre of the upper lip and between the two upper central incisor teeth. This attachment can cause a large gap known as a diastema between the two upper central incisors. It can also cause gingival recession by pulling the gingiva off the bone. Patients who wear dentures can experience problems with retention because, when the lips are moved, the frenulum pulls and will loosen the denture. This can make denture wearing difficult and uncomfortable; having a labial frenectomy will therefore aid the wearing of an upper denture. Patients receiving orthodontic treatment can often have a labial frenectomy to help close the gap between the two front teeth. When a labial frenulum is removed, it will not cause any adverse effects to the lip and mouth.

Procedure

Irrespective of whether a labial or a lingual frenectomy is performed, the procedure involves the freeing of the attachment and is a reasonably straightforward surgical procedure. The maxiollofacial surgeon would explain the procedure to the patient and answer any questions that they may have. Consent would be taken and a local anaesthetic administered. Once the patient is numb, an incision would be made to the attached frenulum to free it using a No. 15 Bard-Parker scalpel blade and handle or a disposable one. A diathermy machine may also be used. A closing suture would be placed using Kilner needle holders, an absorbable suture, Gillie's tissue dissecting forceps, Kilner cheek retractor and long-nosed scissors. The role of the dental nurse and post-operative instructions would be the same as for any other surgical procedure.

For a child under 6 months, tongue-tie release referral is usually made by a paediatrician, midwife or health visitor as indicated by the baby or baby's mother struggling with breast feeding. The procedure requires:

- Consent from parent.
- Topical anaesthetic.
- McIndoe scissors.
- Gauze.

APICECTOMY

An apicectomy comes under the umbrella of endodontic treatments. They are performed by general dental practitioners and endodontists, and are quite often undertaken by maxillofacial surgeons as they are classified as a surgical procedure. When an apicectomy is carried out it involves the removal of the apical third of a tooth which is prepared and filled, ensuring that the apex is completely sealed. The procedure can take up to an hour and a half to complete, depending upon the shape and size of the root canals. Due to this lengthy treatment time, some patients opt for a form of sedation in conjunction with local anaesthetic. Anterior teeth do not take as long to treat as pre-molar and molar teeth. There are various reasons why patients are offered an apicectomy:

- When conventional root canal therapy has failed.
- The root canals of a tooth are narrow or curved.
- An inaccessible canal.
- Escape of an irritant through the apex.
- Persistent infection.
- The tooth has a crown or forms part of a bridge.

Before an apicectomy can be performed the patient would attend a consultation appointment with the maxillofacial surgeon. At this appointment, a medical, dental and social history would be taken. Radiographs would be taken, the intended procedure discussed and consent taken.

Procedure

The patient is settled in the dental chair and provided with personal protective equipment. The maxillofacial surgeon will re-check the status of their medical history and ensure consent is in place and still valid. A brief explanation of the procedure is provided. For pain and anxiety control, topical anaesthetic might be placed prior to the administration of the local anaesthetic. The patient is constantly monitored and reassured.

TRAUMA AND COMPLEX PROCEDURES

The area surrounding the tooth is checked to ensure that it is numb. Once the maxillofacial surgeon is happy that the local anaesthetic is active they will make an incision in the gingiva surrounding the apex of the tooth with a No. 15 Bard-Parker scalpel blade. A gingival flap is raised using either a Mitchell's trimmer or a Howarth's periosteal elevator. The flap is retracted with an Austin's tissue retractor to aid visibility and make it easier for the maxillofacial surgeon to use the straight surgical hand-piece.

The area of infection is identified. The maxillofacial surgeon makes a small hole within the bone with a small rosehead surgical bur placed in a straight surgical hand-piece with an irrigation tube containing 0.9% sodium chloride solution. Some maxillofacial surgeons may choose to use a retrograde hand-piece. The maxillofacial surgeon then amputates the infected root tip (apical third) with the straight surgical hand-piece and bur. Once removed, the area is irrigated with either 0.9% sodium chloride solution in a sterile disposable syringe or chlorhexidine gluconate to remove debris, bacteria and any excess blood present. Any infection is curetted using a curette.

Once free of infection, moisture control must be achieved; cotton wool pellets or ribbon gauze is placed into the prepared area. On occasions bone wax is added to the area. Once effective moisture control has been achieved, Pro-root MTA is mixed and placed using a flat plastic. Any excess cement is removed by irrigating the area. The flap is then sutured back into place using Kilner needle holders, an absorbable suture, Gillie's tissue dissecting forceps, a Kilner cheek retractor and long pointed scissors. Finally, an X-ray is taken to ensure complete filling of the area has been achieved.

The patient is given post-operative care instructions and a review appointment for approximately 3 months, where a further X-ray will be taken to ensure the site has healed. If the patient experiences problems before this appointment, they are requested to return.

ALVEOLECTOMY

An alveolectomy is where a portion of the tooth socket or ridge is surgically removed due to bony irregularities, undercuts and sharp edentulous ridges being present. By performing an alveolectomy, these are reduced and smoothed to allow the insertion and wearing of dentures.

Procedure

The patient is settled in the dental chair and provided with personal protective equipment. The maxillofacial surgeon will re-check the status of their medical history and ensure consent is in place and still valid. A brief explanation of the procedure is provided. For pain and anxiety control topical anaesthetic might be placed prior to the administration of the local anaesthetic. The patient is constantly monitored and reassured. The anaesthetised area and its surrounding are checked to ensure that they is numb. Once the maxillofacial surgeon is happy that the local anaesthetic is active, they will make an incision in the gingiva in the areas where the alveolar ridges are uneven with a No. 15 Bard Parker scalpel blade. A muco-periosteal flap is raised using either a Mitchell's trimmer or a Howarth's periosteal elevator. The maxillofacial surgeon will use a large rosehead surgical bur placed in a straight surgical hand-piece, with an irrigation tube containing 0.9% sodium chloride solution attached, to trim and smooth the bone.

Once the maxillofacial surgeon has undertaken this the ridges are irrigated with 0.9% sodium chloride solution in a sterile syringe. Once all the debris has been removed, the flap is sutured back into place using Kilner needle holders, an absorbable suture, Gillie's tissue dissecting forceps, a Kilner cheek retractor and long pointed scissors. The patient is given post-operative care instructions and a date for a review appointment.

AVULSION

Avulsion occurs when a tooth has received a blow through trauma and becomes detached from its socket within the alveolar bone. If avulsion occurs to a permanent tooth it can be replanted; if a deciduous tooth is however avulsed they are not replaced as they can become infected and interfere with the development of the permanent teeth. If a tooth is avulsed completely and replaced within an hour of the injury taking place, it can be permanently retained in the dental arch. The longer the tooth is absent from its socket, the lower the retention rate once re-implanted.

Advice to patients

In the event of avulsion occurring, patients should be advised:

- To contact the maxillofacial team as soon as possible following any trauma or injury to the teeth or jaws. They can also attend their own general dental practitioner.
- Not to panic. If the tooth is intact and a permanent tooth, carefully pick it up by the crown.
- If the tooth looks fairly clean, not to do any further cleaning. If however it is contaminated with dirt, wash it gently under the cold water tap for approximately 10 seconds. Do not scrub it or clean it with a disinfectant.

TRAUMA AND COMPLEX PROCEDURES

- Continue holding the tooth by its crown and carefully push it back into the socket. If undertaken quickly, the person should not feel any pain. Once in position, the person should bite down on a clean cloth to hold the tooth in place.
- If there is no-one available who is prepared to replant the tooth in its socket, it should be placed in some milk or held in the mouth between the molar teeth and the cheek.
- The person must be taken immediately to a maxillofacial unit or general dental practitioner.
- The tooth should not be allowed to dry out.

Treatment

Upon arrival the patient must be reassured and monitored. The maxillofacial surgeon will explore the circumstances surrounding the avulsion. Consent will be taken, along with the patient's medical history being updated. The tooth will be left *in situ* and cleaned off with either saline, chlorohexidine gluconate or the water from the 3 in 1 tip. Any lacerations will be sutured. An X-ray will be taken to establish if the tooth has been replanted in the correct position. A flexible splint will be placed and antibiotics prescribed. The patient will be given an appointment to return within 7–10 days for root canal therapy treatment to commence and provided with the following care instructions:

- Brush their teeth as normal, twice a day, using a pea-sized amount of toothpaste after eating using a soft headed brush, waiting at least 20 minutes after completion of their meal before doing so.
- Avoid playing any contact sport.
- Eat soft foods.
- Use a fluoride or chlorhexidine gluconate (0.1%) mouthwash.

The splint will eventually be removed, root canal therapy completed and the tooth kept under review periodically both clinically and radiographically.

ROLE OF DENTAL NURSE IN COMPLEX PROCEDURES

The dental nurse will prepare the surgery prior to the patient's arrival and ensure that all equipment is functioning correctly. They will carry out comprehensive infection control by disinfecting the primary and secondary zones and ensure that all instruments, materials and medicaments required for the planned surgical procedure are sterile. They will collect the patient's notes or ensure they are ready on the computer and display the radiographs. They will

TRAUMA AND COMPLEX PROCEDURES

note the patient's medical history to establish if there are any special requirements for the patient and check that consent has been taken. The dental nurse
will collect the patient from the waiting room, checking that they have the correct patient and introduce themselves. They will ask them if they have eaten
and adhered to the pre-operative instructions provided at the last appointment
and if they have any medication they would like placed on the work surface.
They will take the patient's coat and belongings and ask them to take a seat in
the dental chair. Once the patient is settled they will apply the personal protective equipment in the form of a bib and glasses, explaining to the patient the
rationale for each.

When requested, they will scrub in readiness to prepare the items
(Figure 7.17) required for the maxillofacial surgeon with the help of a circulation nurse. The role of a circulation nurse is to open and drop items required
onto a designated surgical field. Throughout the procedure, constant aspiration
and retraction of soft tissues, as required, will take place. Instruments will
be passed at the correct stage of the procedure, ensuring a sterile field. If
applicable, the dental nurse will hold a retractor. Continual reassurance and
monitoring of the patient's vital signs will be undertaken. The maxillofacial
surgeon may request the dental nurse to cut the sutures when being placed.

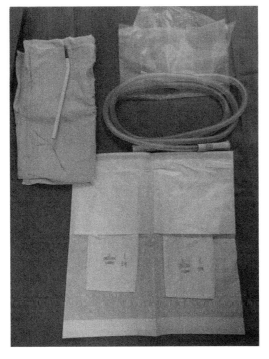

Figure 7.17 Sterile surgical gloves, sterile drape and sterile suction tubing and tip.

TRAUMA AND COMPLEX PROCEDURES

They will also ensure excellent cross-infection control and the health and safety of all. If requested, the dental nurse may provide verbal and written post-operative care instructions.

Once the patient has left they will dispose of the waste correctly and carry out infection control procedures in the form of disinfection and sterilisation, returning the patient's notes and radiographs to file. They may be required to make further appointments. When assisting with biopsies, the dental nurse will ensure that the pathology laboratory sheet is correctly completed and the sample is dispatched to the pathology laboratory. When assisting with an apicectomy, they will mix the Pro-root MTA and process the X-rays. Before assisting with implants, it is beneficial for the dental nurse to undertake some form of training due to the complex equipment used.

Index

Basic Guide to Oral and Maxillofacial Surgery, First Edition. Nicola Rogers and Cinzia Pickett.
© 2017 John Wiley & Sons Ltd. Published 2017 by John Wiley & Sons Ltd.

Printed and bound by CPI Group (UK) Ltd, Croydon, CR0 4YY
18/08/2022
03142567-0001